The Art in Personal Training

Using Martial Art Techniques in Personal Training

By Charles "Charlie" Spence, Jr.

ISBN: 9781696974783

Table of Contents

Preface

"And Jesus increased in wisdom and stature, and in favor with God and men" (Luke 2:52).

For a long time, I have been intrigued by this passage of scripture. The passage is very telling about the expectations God has for every person. Jesus demonstrated absolute human perfection. He increased four basic components that should characterize every human being: mental, physical, spiritual, and social. God designed human beings to be able to function in these four areas if they are to live long, happy, and quality lives. Since that is the case, I wanted to know what God wants humanity to do to meet these expectations.

Being physically fit plays a vital role in a person's overall well-being. Satan understood this when he approached God concerning Job's spiritual attachment to God. Satan accused Job of worshiping God for nothing because God showed Job favor by protecting him from difficulty and trouble (Job 1:9-11). Ultimately, Satan believed that a man would give everything for his physical well-being. Satan insisted that if Job suffered physically, such would affect him spiritually (Job 2:4-5). Satan knows human behavior since he has observed man for a long time (Job 1:6-7). Physical infirmities also affected men and women socially. Many of the prominent folk in Jesus' day did not think those suffering from disease or physical maladies as worthy of inclusion or being able to socialize freely (Luke 13:10-17, John 9). Leprosy in Bible times was debilitating and resulted in social isolation (Lev. 13:45-46; Num. 5:1-4). Because Jesus knew the social stigma that sickness and disease brought upon man, He demonstrated a deep concern for man's physical welfare through healing (Mark 1:40-42, Matt. 9:35-37).

The Lord provides knowledge that all may be wise as to how one can achieve physical fitness. He lets us know that He has high regard for the human body, and so should we when he says, *"Or do you not know that your body is a temple of the Holy Spirit who is in you, whom you have from God, and that you are not your own? For you have been bought with a price: therefore, glorify God in your body"* (1 Cor. 6:19-20). God wants people to present their bodies as holy and acceptable unto Him (Rom. 12:1). Even God's people are concerned for the health and wellbeing of humanity (3 John 2). The Lord wants us to see the value in exercise (1 Tim 4:8) and proper nutrition (Pro. 23:20). Whatever a person does regarding exercise and food, such must bring glory to God (1 Cor. 10:31).

For this reason, I chose to get into personal fitness training. I look at this as a part of a ministry to help men and women achieve the glory that God intended. I want to take the years of knowledge with which God has blessed me to work with people of all ages and fitness levels to help them *"increase in wisdom and stature and in favor with God and with man."* To extend this work beyond the borders of my immediate community, I write this book.

Paul alluded to fighting in such a way as to discipline his body (1 Cor. 9:26-27) effectively. So, I want to incorporate twenty-two years of my martial art training to help many people discipline their bodies. I will help others realize that this journey will not be easy but will yield great rewards and ultimately transform people's lives (Heb. 12:11-13).

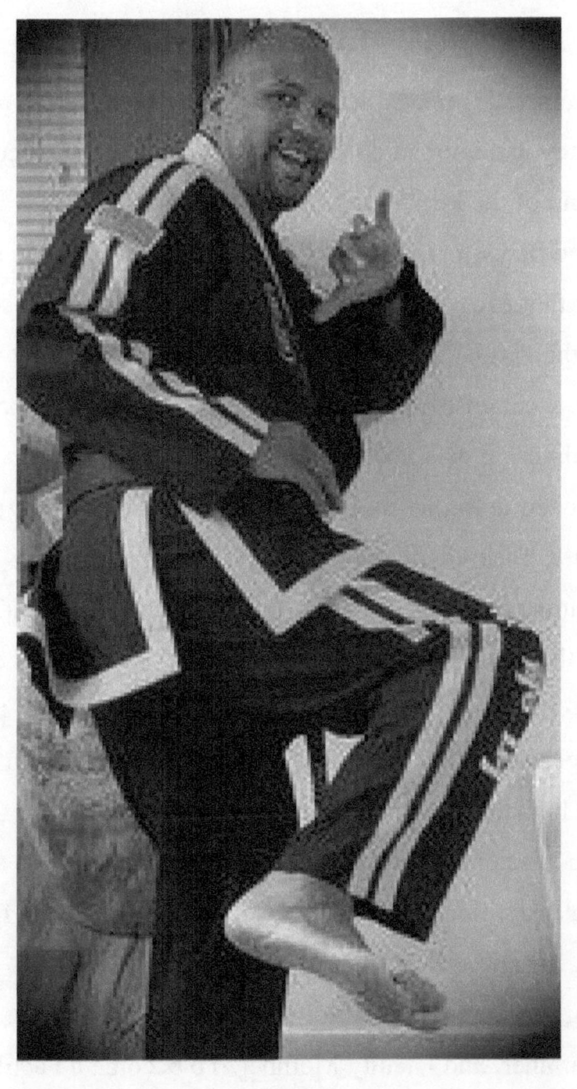

Introduction

As a personal trainer, I have had clients interested in attaining whatever fitness goals they had but had concerns about the routines becoming mundane. I realized that one of the keys to a personal trainer's success is maintaining client adherence to the fitness programs. I did not want to simply use the same tried and tested routines that every personal trainer uses. While a good trainer can modify the uses of all the various exercise equipment, machines, and even a client's body weight, to keep exercise programs exciting, I wanted to have a whole new approach to delivering personal training.

I had been doing martial arts on and off since I was seven years old. I practiced Karate, Taekwondo, and Kung Fu well into my mid-30s. At the age of 35, I began training in the martial art of Choi Kwang Do. Grand Master Choi was the founder of this art in 1987. Grand Master Choi (GMC) was one of the original masters of Taekwondo (TKD). By the age of 30, GMC's TKD training took a toll on his body because of the harsh and lock-out movements in TKD techniques. After studying human anatomy, kinesiology, and biomechanics, GMC developed an art based upon scientific principles that proved effective as a self-defense tool and a way for practitioners to achieve optimal health and fitness. Many had dubbed the organization "The Martial Art for Life."

During my tenure at Choi Kwang Do, I became an International Instructor, Examiner, and Faculty Member. To become a Faculty Member, I had to take more extensive courses than anything that I had to take to certify as a Personal Trainer. I studied anatomy, kinesiology, biomechanics, psychology, and applied science. This was on top of the detailed instruction in all the pillars (which are 10) of CKD. I eventually became a 6th degree International Master Instructor. I built a successful martial art school in Lithonia, Georgia. I had as many as 178 students and a staff of 24 instructors. During that time, I developed programs that helped the students to be able to defend themselves. I also focused on health and fitness assessments that allowed me to tailor programs specific to children, teens, adults, and seniors' fitness levels. Because of my knowledge in applied science, I was also able to tailor my martial art classes to accommodate those struggling with symptomologies of various degenerative conditions, obesity, PTSD, ADD, ADHD, and autism. Those that were once prohibited from participating in such activities due to the previously mentioned problems can now go on to lead productive lives through their participation in our martial art program.

The techniques help to keep the training interesting. I had a good-sized staff that taught various classes in my school. This provided variety to the students as each instructor had a personality that they brought to the way each delivered the instruction. While the techniques were the same, the instructors did not teach them in the same way. This made each class unique—the very nature of the martial art program provided variety. Every two months, a student can test for belt promotion. The student learns new techniques, patterns, and drills with each new belt. In personal training, 6-8 weeks of consistent training helps the client master the program, allowing the client to move to the next level. This helps to avoid plateauing and maintain adherence to the fitness program. In an industry that emphasizes goal setting, incorporating martial art techniques in the training programs will give the client more to look forward. As was the case with my students in my martial art school, so it is with my training clients. They are anxious to learn what new techniques and drills they will learn next.

The martial art techniques that I incorporate in my training programs are those I use for myself to stay fit. To be healthy, a person needs to have cardiovascular fitness, muscular strength, endurance, and as close to the full range of motion (flexibility). Therefore, I believe that martial arts have a place in personal training, and I will continue to incorporate martial arts in fitness programs for my clients that want to break away from the mundane.

After December 2018, Choi Kwang Do Martial Art International went in a different direction that compromised its ability to deliver safe and practical training to its students. As a result, many schools have pulled away, including mine. We are now a part of the newly formed Universal Martial Art (UMA). My school in Arizona is Spence Martial Art Academy or SMART Academy. We have not abandoned the principles upon which CKD had been established. We practice the same curriculum, techniques, and drills. These are just as effective for health and fitness. Not only do we embrace being the "Martial Art for Life," we are the "Martial Art for everyone!"

This book explains personal training and its benefits. It develops why martial arts have a role to play in effective personal training. It details the effectiveness of the techniques themselves. It also details the impact martial arts have on disease prevention and relief. The book addresses how this approach to personal training impacts various populations. And while some may think personal training is enough for health and fitness, the book briefly addresses food and nutrition.

I hope that many will read this book with the intent of wanting to be healthy and fit. Bear in mind that reading this book will not turn you into the wellness picture that most only dream of; you will have to act upon and do the things outlined in this book.

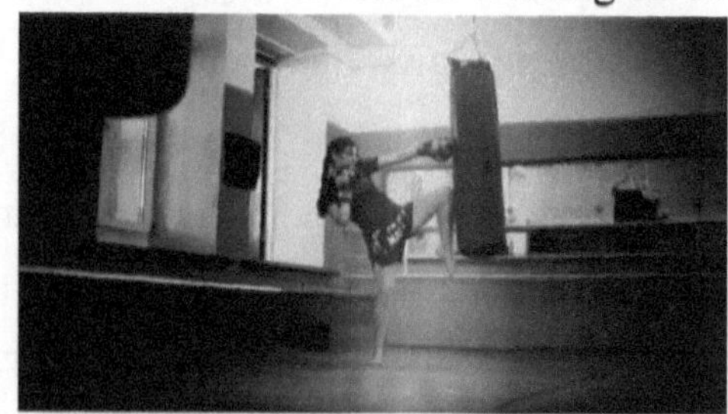

Personal Training

We live in an age when many citizens of the United States are struggling with their weight, fitness, and overall health. According to the Centers for Disease Control and Prevention, a 2015-2016 National Center for Health Statistics determined that 71.6% of adults over 20 years of age are obese or overweight. The stats do not fare better with children. On average, 14.3% of kids between 2 and 19 are obese. The problem is not just with obesity. Obesity can lead to various debilitating and degenerative health conditions. Obesity is usually a suspect in cardiovascular disease, hypertension, back pain, and type 2 diabetes, just to name a few. It is mindboggling that obesity is one of the most preventable health disorders, yet most people choose not to prevent it.

In a November 2015 article written by Adda Bjarnadottir, she cites nine reasons obesity is not a choice. She talks of gut bacteria, food addiction, infancy and childhood nutritional habits, genetics, education, hormones, etc. While many of these or a combination of these may impact a person's body composition, can these be why 84% of the United States population are obese? I believe a person can make wise and healthy choices regarding health and nutrition. It is as simple as having an egg instead of a donut for breakfast or tuna on whole wheat instead of a Big Mac for lunch.

Weight gain or weight loss is determined by the number of calories ingested versus the number expended. If a person wants to lose 1 to 2 pounds a week, they must reduce their caloric intake by 3500 to 7000 calories a week or 500-1000 calories a day. The formula for calculating caloric needs is simple. Multiply your current weight by 15, which would be the number of calories you must consume to sustain that weight. To gain 1 pound, one must consume 3500 more calories than the body needs; to lose 1 pound, you must consume 3500 calories less. While there are instances where genetics or hormones may play a role in obesity, caloric intake, and lifestyle management determine the body's composition. I agree with Ms. Bjarnadottir's point: obesity can result from a lack of education. When it comes to health and fitness, education is a valuable tool.

Many do not know the impact that poor nutritional choices have on their health and wellness. They do not see the effect that exercise has on their well-being. Today, we are witnessing the consequences of removing recess and physical education from school activities and curriculums. More channels on the TV keep more people on the couch. Kids would rather play sports on XBOX than play them outside. Physical activity has diminished while sedentary living has increased. Someone must sound the alarm so people know that they are endangering the quality of their lives with their lifestyle choices. That is the reason I got into personal training. I want to be one of those that sound the alarm. I want to educate people on the impact of lifestyle choices on health and fitness. I want to see people improve the quality of their lives, live longer and be happy. As an ACE-certified personal trainer, I have the education and knowledge necessary to provide safe and practical fitness routines for individuals of all ages. I will initially meet with the client to determine their fitness goals. As a personal trainer, I will help the client establish SMART goals.

- Specific
- Measurable
- Attainable
- Realistic
- Time-based

I will ensure that the clients get the right program tailored to those specific goals. I will also monitor the performance of those exercises so that the clients perform them correctly and safely and that those exercises are effective in helping them attain their goals.

Fighting to Be Fit

I am sure that most people have noticed over the years that boxers are some of the best-conditioned athletes in the world. Their training consists of 5 days of training for 3-5 hours each day. This they do to be able to fight effectively for twelve 3-minute rounds. This comprises a total of 36 minutes of fighting.

Boxing is an anaerobic activity. Anaerobic means "without oxygen." This kind of activity can only be sustained for brief periods. The anaerobic movements consist of powerful bursts of speed and strength. Anaerobic training is high-intensity training. To be most effective, this type of training must be done in intervals. It effectively burns a significant number of calories during the workout sessions. Yet, the same activity burns calories even after the workout is completed as an additional benefit. This is "afterburn." More technically, it is exercise post-exercise oxygen consumption or EPOC. Anaerobic training produces an oxygen deficit and a need for more energy. The body stores energy in glycogen (a more complex form of glucose) in the muscles. When the body struggles to get oxygen, the muscles deplete themselves of glycogen resulting in the body being tired and a burn or soreness in the muscles (lactic acid buildup). After a workout, to build up oxygen reserves and aid in recovery, the body must burn more energy (calories). Thus, anaerobic training is effective for weight loss, even at rest.

Boxers usually have very little body fat and are muscular, well-toned, and defined. This they do without incorporating a weightlifting program. They often use their body weight in variable movements and rely upon resistance training with heavy bags, speed bags and focus mitts. They use their power to strike these objects, triggering a muscular response. This creates lean muscle mass and the muscles' cut or definition while improving muscular endurance and strength.

In the last twenty years, a new fighting style has emerged on the scene: mixed martial arts. The training is just as intense as boxing, if not more so, to stay competitive in the matches. The Ultimate Fighting Championship originated back in 1993, in which fighters representing a wide range of fighting styles competed against each other. After a few years, the UFC fighting style became very popular with those interested in fitness. Many health clubs and fitness boutiques have adopted the MMA or UFC style of training as a form of fitness training.

Years before UFC made its mark in the sports and fitness world; Billy Blanks arrived on the scene with his Tae Bo workout. After developing this fitness regimen using martial art techniques, he began working with celebrities and eventually produced videos that helped transform people's fitness lifestyles.

Universal Martial Art (UMA) techniques are based upon scientific principles that work with the human body's natural movement. This makes the use of UMA safe and effective. The movements, when combined, form patterns and speed drills that produce aerobic activity. When the practitioner performs the patterns and speed drills faster, this creates anaerobic exercise. The practitioner conducts the techniques on shields, heavy bags, and focus mitts. This provides the resistance training needed for muscular strength, endurance, tone, and growth. Incorporating these techniques into a personal training program will benefit cardiovascular health, muscular strength, and flexibility. Unlike boxing and MMA-type fighting and training, there is no sparing or contact with UMA training. So, it is safe and non-competitive and people of all ages and fitness levels can participate in and benefit from any personal training that incorporates the UMA techniques. Also, unlike Billy Blanks' Tae Bo, which is based upon Tae

Kwon Do and Karate methodologies, the movements in UMA are not stressful. UMA does not lock out any of the kicks, strikes, or punches, making is easier on the joints and ligaments.

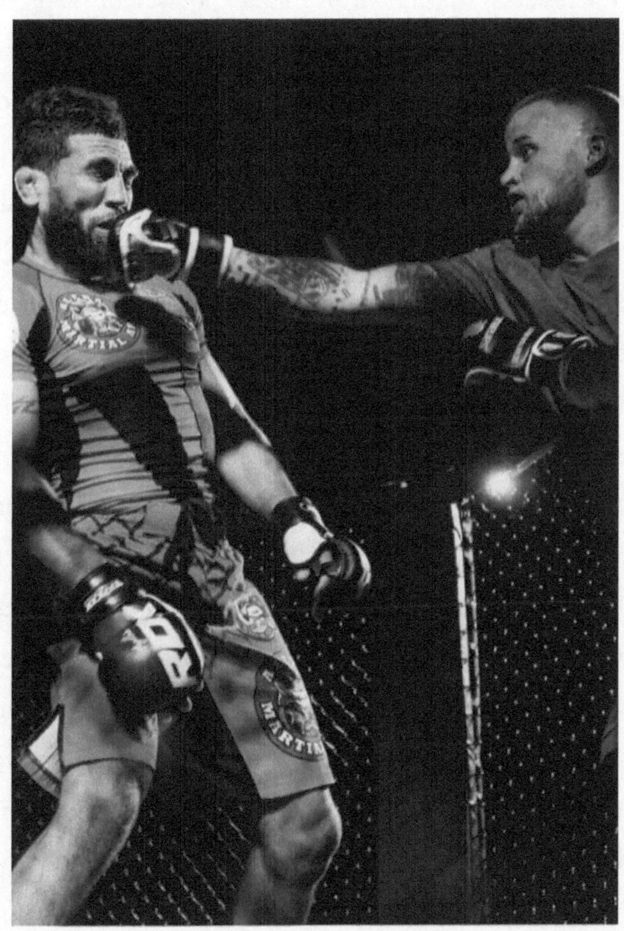

Martial Arts in Personal Training

I am a nationally recognized certified personal trainer; I am also a 6th Degree Black Belt, International Chief instructor, and Examiner in Universal Martial Art. Universal Martial Art is based upon scientific principles of anatomy, kinesiology, biomechanics, and psychology. These are the same principles that every Personal Trainer must learn to be an effective certified personal trainer. Universal Martial Art is effective as a self-defense system; it is also effective in promoting optimal health. Universal Martial Art will aid in cardiovascular fitness, muscular strength and definition, and flexibility when one performs it frequently. Each basic technique involves the total body. It triggers the kinetic chain in which each movement of a hand, arm, leg, or foot affects other parts of the body. This involves skeletal, muscular, and even psychological aspects of human fitness. The movements (blocking, punching, and kicking) can be combined into patterns that the practitioner can perform aerobically or anaerobically. Increased cardiovascular fitness will result in weight loss, increased functionality, and greater endurance. When the practitioner performs those techniques during bag or shield work, they are involved in resistance training. Resistance training helps to improve muscle strength and endurance. Each movement, along with the Universal Martial Art stretches, helps to improve range of motion or flexibility.

Using Universal Martial Art to achieve physical fitness is a highly effective tool. My clients not only find it effective but also fun and rewarding. This is something that people of all ages can utilize as it is safe, does not require weights or any such equipment, and does not require a gym membership.

Universal Martial Art Techniques and Personal Training

If done correctly, Universal Martial Art (UMA) techniques will provide an excellent self-defense model and provide a means of achieving optimum health for the practitioner. This is because of the mechanics of the movements involved in performing the basic techniques. For UMA techniques to be effective, the student must complete every element of performing the movement correctly. Every technique utilizes sequential movement. This promotes the fluidity of motion when performing the techniques. The UMA technique is the sum of all its parts. The student must perform each part properly for the technique to be effective. This one does by using the Kinetic (production of movement) Chain.

The kinetic chain consists of the skeletal, muscular, and nervous systems. When the elements that make up the kinetic chain are operating correctly, force maximization should be the result. UMA techniques are designed to utilize the kinetic chain. As the student performs the techniques, he will dramatically affect the nervous system. In UMA, the nervous system is conditioned to respond a certain way with the techniques performed. The student can eventually perform the techniques without giving much thought to the elements of movement that generate the force of those techniques that they perform. This is much like walking or running. A person usually does not give much thought to all the elements that make up walking.

The UMA movements are natural, and thus people of all ages can effectively perform them. If the student does not utilize every element that makes up the kinetic chain properly, he can harm his body. The human body responds to unnatural movement or a force exerted upon it that it has not been used to. The muscles, joints, and ligaments send messages to the brain that indicate discomfort or pain. It is as if the muscles themselves have their little brains. The information that the brain gathers from the output of the muscles and the responses that the muscles' responses to the stimuli exerted upon them, which experts call proprioception. This process helps determine the amount of effort necessary for the body to move efficiently. In addition, what is amazing, this process accounts for an awareness of how the condition of each limb of the body concerns each other. So, when a student develops to the point of effectively performing the UMA techniques, his body will respond favorably to his movements.

This leads to neuromuscular efficiency. When the student achieves such, the result would be speed and power. Just performing the movements properly is not enough, however. The practitioner must align his body correctly. The stances must be balanced and aligned for the student to perform the techniques correctly. UMA stances, when done properly, help generate the necessary speed and power in performing the techniques. UMA incorporates dynamic stances, which are required to accommodate the proper execution of many of the techniques. Dynamics in physics refers to force, energy, or power. Simply defined, it is accelerated movement. From UMA dynamic stances, the student can effectively move in response to the conditions upon him. This helps make UMA so unique to more traditional martial art styles.

The way a student trains in UMA is the way that student is expected to fight if the need arises. We call this positive transfer. Most traditional martial art styles result in a negative transfer. Again, what makes UMA so unique is its impact on the nervous system. If he were to fight, the traditional martial artist would have to adapt to the conditions in a way that would be detrimental to his entire body. Think of the stress that builds up within a body that one has not adequately conditioned to deal with certain stimuli that come its way. The mechanics of UMA techniques, from start to finish, were designed to meet the needs of responding to the stimuli that comes the body's way efficiently. We call this functional efficiency. When the student practices UMA techniques in the air, he performs them fluidly and without locking out the joints. In other words, the student performs the movement following through the point of contact. Utilizing the kinetic chain, the student produces the force (speed and power) necessary to shock its target. However, when performed in the air, there is a point where the student must decelerate the technique. This will undoubtedly mimic the movement necessary to strike a target. However, without resistance, the student must know to decelerate the strike. When traditional martial art techniques are performed, such often results in injury to the body because the force that the practitioner generates to stop the strike, rather than simply decelerate, transfers back to the body.

Another benefit of utilizing UMA techniques is the ability to equally train both sides of the body. In the case of an attack, the student will be able to defend himself no matter what direction the attack is coming from. This is because the student's continuous performance of the techniques positively impacts the central nervous system (CNS). Once again, the student is conditioned to address the external stimuli in a stress-free and balanced way. As mentioned earlier, performing the UMA techniques can lead to optimum health and well-being. The student will be able to maximize and work through his range of motion. This would result in the body staving off muscle and bone deterioration, aches, and pains. Even performing the UMA blocks will go a long way in strengthening the human body's core. All UMA movements work through the core. When the core, which is made up of the area around the trunk and pelvis, is strong, such will go a long way in preventing injury and maximizing overall good health. The core is the center of gravity in the body. If the core is weak, such will affect posture and lead to back pain and muscle injuries. Many in the martial arts world do not understand the process by which one can achieve optimum neuromuscular efficiency. This is because traditional martial arts are not rooted in scientific principles. UMA employs biomechanics, plyometrics, anatomy, kinesiology, and physiology. These systems which operate within the human body must work together to achieve overall efficiency. In traditional martial arts, they have not studied the impact the sequence of their movements has on the human body to make it perform more efficiently. This they do in sports like golf, bowling, and baseball. The athlete must perform a sequence of movements to respond to the event to achieve maximum efficiency. When he fails to do this, such will result in inefficiency and even injury.

Therefore, UMA is unique and unequaled in the martial arts world. This art is not simply concerned with the "appearance" of generating power but rather efficiency in generating that power. This art is concerned with achieving and maintaining optimum health and well-being. To do so, the student must practice and perform every technique properly. The student will benefit immensely from such training physically and mentally. Mentally, he will feel confident knowing he can execute the techniques necessary to defend himself in a fluid and almost reflexive manner because he would have conditioned his nervous system to respond that way.

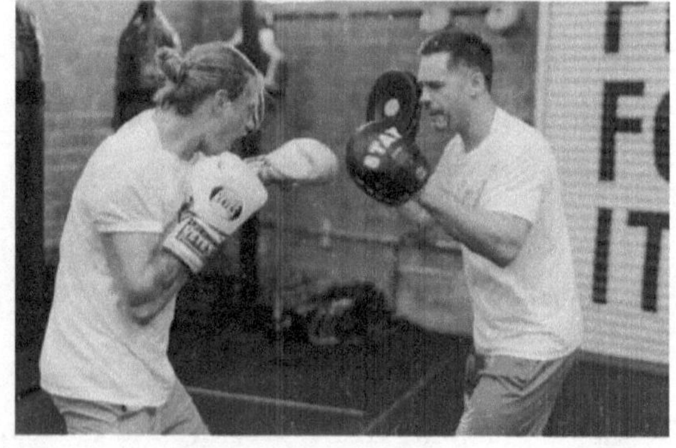

Personal Training and Aerobic Activity

Aerobics (with oxygen) or "Cardio," in modern-day fitness vernacular, is a physical activity that has the amount of intensity to increase breathing, heart rate, and blood flow for a sustained period that is longer than a few minutes. The increased breathing is to bring oxygen into the lungs. From the lungs, it goes into the blood and the heart. The heart pumps the oxygenated blood to the tissues, muscles, and organs from the heart. Muscle movement creates an oxygen demand. The greater the movement (intensity, duration, and frequency), the greater the oxygen demand. Aerobic activity is more than everyday activities: walking from place to place, sitting, reading, cooking, etc. These activities do not usually raise one's heart rate and breathing.

Along with oxygen, the heart pumps all the nutrients that the body needs to maintain proper health and fitness. Oxygen in the muscles is vital for energy production upon which the muscles feed. Oxygen helps to turn carbohydrates and fats into energy. Aerobic exercise usually burns more fat over an extended period than carbs because fat is denser. There are nine calories per gram of fat instead of 4 grams of carbohydrates. Regular aerobic exercise leads to muscular efficiency and cardiovascular health. The lungs will have greater capacity, the heart will not have to beat as fast, and one will experience greater endurance. Some of the benefits of aerobic exercise are:

- Weight loss
- Endurance
- Disease prevention
- Better mood
- Increased Energy
- Stronger heart
- Brain efficiency

- Lessen stress
- It helps regulate blood sugar
- Increases performance

Personal trainers are aware of the benefits of aerobic training and look to incorporate such into any personal training program for clients. This, accompanied by anaerobic and resistance training sessions, will promote optimal health and fitness.

Martial Arts and Aerobic Activity

Since aerobic activity requires muscle movement at a level of intensity that increases breathing and heart rate sustained for more than a few minutes, incorporating martial art techniques would help do that. The martial art techniques in Universal Martial Art (UMA) are biomechanically sound, providing safe and effective movement to produce aerobic activity. Universal Martial Art utilizes blocks, strikes, punches, and kicks in its program. The movements involve contracting and expanding the muscles with some velocity to increase oxygen delivery to the active area. The practitioner can engage in a total body workout by combining the various techniques and increasing aerobic capacity. The practitioner can control the intensity, duration, and frequency when they do the training independently.

One of the benefits of incorporating martial arts into personal training for aerobic activity is that it does not require any machines or equipment. Thus, the practitioner can perform the martial art routine anywhere and anytime. Compared to other aerobic activities that one can freely do without machines or equipment, such as walking, martial arts provide the practitioner with:

- A full-body workout – the combined martial arts techniques affect every body part.
- Better posture and balance – martial arts, especially Universal Martial Art, focus on proper technique and movement based on biomechanics and kinesiology.
- Greater stamina and endurance – the oxygen demand that comes from the practitioner using total body movement is better at improving cardiovascular fitness.
- Better reaction times – something that a practitioner will not be able to develop doing any other kind of aerobic activity.

These benefits alone are enough to encourage fitness-minded people to find personal trainers that utilize martial arts in their fitness programs. More personal trainers should learn martial arts to create variety in their fitness programs.

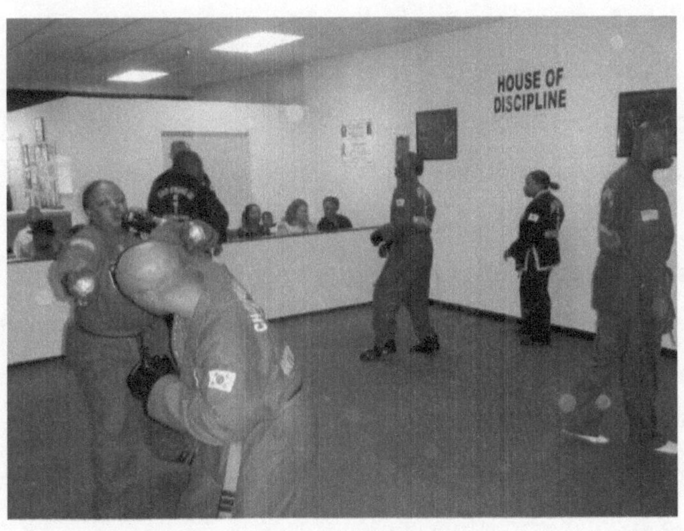

Personal Training and Anaerobic Activity

Anaerobic (without oxygen) activity involves exercise or movement performed at a level of intensity that the cardiovascular system cannot deliver oxygen to the muscles fast enough to sustain the activity. The practitioner is out of breath with such exercise, usually less than 2 minutes. The critical determinant that catapults the practitioner into anaerobic activity is the intensity of the workout. Usually, the exercises that one performs anaerobically require a short burst of intense energy. The activity helps to break down glucose without oxygen.

Consequently, anaerobic activity will help burn more calories after exercise because of the oxygen demands of the muscles involved in the workout. Anaerobic activity demands more energy than the Aerobic system can produce. This triggers the body to convert energy from stored sources in the body to those working muscles. Enough glucose is stored in the muscles to accommodate short bursts of intense activity. Once those stores are depleted, there is a lactic acid or muscle burn buildup. The muscle burn is not a buildup of lactate but rather lactate production. The burn or soreness is the body's way of forcing the cessation of strenuous activity to promote recovery.

The benefits of anaerobic activity are increased stamina and endurance, strength, and VO2 max improvement. VO2 max is the amount of oxygen the body can convert to energy. When there is not enough oxygen, the muscles use lactate to aid in restoring energy. A person performing the anaerobic exercise will only be able to exercise for a brief period, usually no more than 2 minutes. When a person exercises between 80% and 90% of their target heart rate zone, they are in anaerobic activity. The body will go into defense mode to prevent injury or damage from the high exertion. The systems needed to trigger muscle contraction slow down to avoid overexertion consequences.

Because of the increased benefits of anaerobic training and the complexity of the exercises associated with such activity, one would need a certified personal trainer to monitor the exercise effectively. The personal trainer will be able to determine that the exercise is safe, beneficial, and adequately measure the client's performance. Personal trainers should use anaerobic exercises in their training programs if they genuinely are concerned about helping their clients reach optimal fitness.

Martial Arts and Anaerobic Training

As mentioned earlier in this book, much of the training for fighting activities, whether boxing or mixed martial arts, uses anaerobic exercises. This is because the practitioner must prepare him or herself to endure several short periods of intense activity. They need to build stamina, speed, and strength. The ideal training for this activity is anaerobic. If training for fighting yields such benefits for competition, could not one train in such a way without the competition and improve fitness and health? When one considers the benefits of fight training, the answer is a definite yes. What are some of the benefits of fight training?

- Aerobic and anaerobic conditioning
- Improved strength in every muscle in the body
- Increased coordination
- Increased speed
- Lean muscle mass
- Mental toughness
- Weight loss

Since many who train for fighting events such as boxing and mixed martial arts are in such top physical condition, it should not be a surprise that performing martial arts for fitness would prove beneficial. Martial art techniques, when performed non-competitively, provide an effective exercise for the practitioner to achieve overall health and fitness. The practitioner can combine martial art techniques to create patterns and speed drills. When the practitioner performs the patterns and speed drills as fast as possible for short periods, the practitioner exercises anaerobically. Because of the complexity of the movements and the use of the total body, martial arts techniques provide the ultimate full-body workout when performed anaerobically. With the added variety and benefit of martial art training, martial arts are an ideal tool in any personal trainer's fitness program.

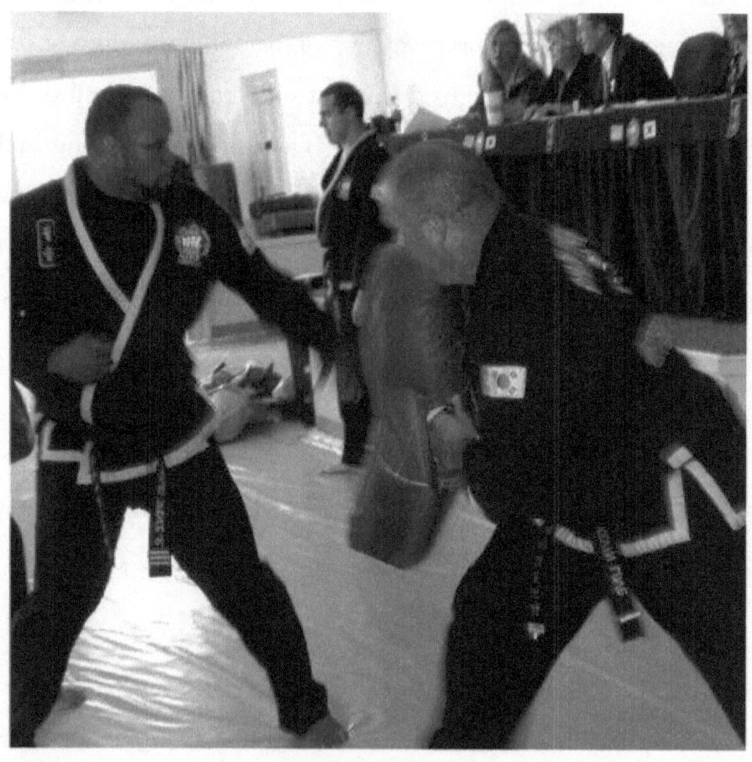

An Analysis of My Personal Training

From a child, I have always been active. I was always involved in athletics as a part of a team. I played football, basketball, and baseball and ran track competitively. In college, I played football. The tendency for many people who have been athletic and now have jobs, many of which are office jobs and require much sitting, is to become sedentary, gain weight, and develop health problems. I do not want to be another statistic. While I may not be involved in competitive sports, I engage in exercise that will keep me fit, strong, flexible, and healthy. Also, because I enjoy life, I want to be around for a long time. In other words, I want to live for as long as I can, being able to do all the things that I want to do physically.

My Exercise Habits

One of the first things I had to realize is that I am not a youth anymore. At the writing of the book, I am 57 years young. My exercise routine must factor that into it. I need to keep up my endurance and stay strong to prevent the onset of arthritis, bone loss, or diminished mobility. I also need to remain flexible to maintain my proper range of motion. With that said, my routine consists of 5 days of exercise each week.

1. Day 1 – (cardio for fat burning) 15 minutes of warm-up and dynamic stretching, 30-45 minutes of cardio at a pace of 750 calories burned an hour. After, I will perform Universal Martial Art patterns at a moderate pace from white belt to my highest pattern at 6th-degree black belt. This takes about 1.25 hours. This is finished with 15 minutes of combined cool down and static stretching.

2. Day 2 – (Endurance and Strength) 15 Minutes of warm-up and dynamic stretching. I perform a weight circuit for major muscle groups. I work larger muscles first (agonist then antagonist), legs, core, back, chest, and arms. In between sets, I perform UMA speed drills as fast as possible for 1 minute and then rest for 2 minutes. This takes about 1.5 hours. I finish with 10 minutes of bag work, then 15 minutes of cool down and static stretching.

3. Day 3 repeats day 1

4. Day 4 repeats day 2

5. Day 5 – HIIT (High Intensity, Interval Training), a real fat burner

Locomotor, Nonlocomotor, and Manipulative Movement in Workout Plans

Locomotor movement is the building block of all movement. Whether walking, running, skipping, or hopping, moving from one place to another is locomotor. This helps to achieve coordination and balance and leads to more complex movement. Nonlocomotor movement is any movement the body does without traveling from one place to another. This involves twisting, bending, stretching, etc. This helps promote the body's full range of motion, posture, and balance. Manipulative movement involves exertion or resistance in movement. It involves kicking, pushing, pulling, throwing, etc. This promotes muscle building and strength for these kinds of activities.

Why I Use Martial Art in My Personal Training

Universal Martial Art incorporates all three areas of movement in its program. Nonlocomotor movement involves performing the basic techniques in the air using sequential movement and twisting of the frame. Locomotor movement becomes necessary to bridge the distance between the attacker and the

UMA practitioner. The student performs this by walking and striking the opponent, sliding toward the opponent with a kick, and using a jumping punch or kick. Manipulative movement involves hitting a target or kicking a target. All these are a part of the workout I do. With tennis, a person utilizes all three. The same is true for swimming. So, I get my share of these types of movements.

Energy Systems Affected by My Workout Plan

Because muscles need energy for movement, a process makes this possible. Muscles do not derive their energy directly from food. The body must convert the food ultimately into Adenosine Triphosphate or ATP. This releases the energy to the muscles in the form of glucose through the delivery system mitochondria. When it is stored in muscle, this is glycogen. Anaerobic exercise taps into ATP, releasing enough energy to sustain up to 80 seconds of high-intensity anaerobic activity. During aerobic activities, the body will rely upon carbohydrates as an immediate energy source. The body produces energy from the chemical reactions that use oxygen. The body needs a constant source of energy. To wait on the metabolizing of fats and complex carbohydrates would take too long to keep all the body's organs functioning properly. So, the body needs an immediate source of energy. During aerobic activity for 20 minutes or longer, the aerobic energy system utilizes fats and proteins to convert to energy, providing energy for extended periods.

The aerobic system needs oxygen to help convert carbohydrates, fats, and proteins into the energy the muscles need for sustained activity. My workout uses both systems. It probably relies more on the anaerobic system. This is by design because I rather have the energy stored in muscle for immediate use rather than stored as fat for later use.

Units of Exercise

With the exercise regimen as described in the beginning, if I commit to doing it consistently, assuming I was out of shape, and I incorporated a balanced nutritional diet, with proper sleep, in 8 weeks, I will have improved cardiovascular fitness, increased aerobic capacity and 16 to 24 pounds of weight loss.

Impact of Exercise

Concerning anaerobic power, the training needs to be at a level that the person can perform. I like HIIT training because it helps to increase my fast-twitch muscle fibers, my ability to tolerate lactate, decrease my recovery time, and lower my resting heart rate.

About aerobic power, the exercise helps increase overall cardiorespiratory fitness, enabling circulation and oxygen flow to produce energy for muscles. It also helps to improve mitochondrial function in the muscles.

Training and Rest Times

Some suggest that people should not exercise for more than three days in a row. I can't entirely agree; providing the exercise is diverse, as with first-day cardio training and next-day strength training. With anaerobic training, one should perform on alternate days because the muscles need to build. I work out four days in a row and have an optional 5th day. My rest periods are fine if I get a good night's sleep when all the regeneration occurs.

Issues with Motor Skills and Learning

One significant issue with the motor skills involved in the workout is developing muscle memory. The brain stores what it needs to control or tell the muscles how to function. This is procedural memory. The problem that can develop from this is that a person performs a task repeatedly but wrong. The brain only knows to inform the muscles how to move for the given task; it does not let the muscles know whether they are performing the task correctly. Children learn tasks and activities by numbers. In Universal Martial Art, each movement has a sequence. The instructor helps the student perform each sequence properly so that when muscle memory sets in, he will do the task correctly.

The person needs to tweak their exercise program from time to time to make it more appealing and not boring. Also, this needs to happen to help avoid the dreaded plateau. Some days I will simply do my patterns one after the other, or I will pyramid the patterns. I will work the same muscles but will change the exercise. Instead of weights, I may do isometric exercises. I have much depth in my exercise regimen and certainly plenty of variety.

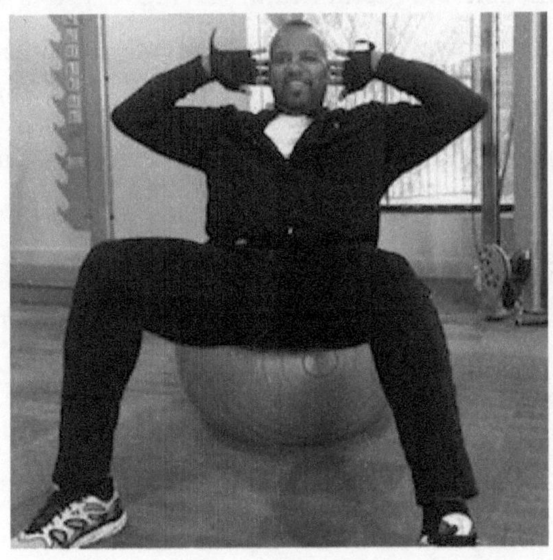

Personal Training for Health, Wellness, Quality of Life

Fitness is an integral part of health and longevity. If it is going to be effective in achieving overall optimum health, a good fitness program should be rooted in scientific evidence and not the latest trends or commercial products. The fitness program's components must include physical exercise, good nutrition, and a sense of well-being from a good mental attitude. Longevity is the desire of many people. While some do live long, the quality of their lives may not have been what they desired. What is the point of living longer if you are not living well? Living long yet remaining physically, mentally, and spiritually healthy is a challenge that requires a strong will and wisdom. A person who desires to live long can receive this wonderful blessing only if he has and utilizes the knowledge and exercise understanding of an anti-aging lifestyle program.

Today many are living to 100 years of age. With advances in science and a greater emphasis on healthy lifestyles, many people are learning to listen to their bodies (from which we get wisdom) and addressing the needs of the body, mind, and soul to accommodate long-term health. Living to 100 is within the grasp of just about everyone. However, the challenge of our time presents a great distraction to the desire of many to live healthy and long: *"The spirit is willing, but the flesh is weak."* Too many succumb to the temptations and tendencies of a sedentary life. Television, video games, computers, and jobs make it easy to procrastinate in the human will to live longer, healthier lives. It is easier and more pleasurable for many to maintain a diet of so-called "comfort foods," which contribute to poor health. When these tendencies take their toll, disease and degenerative conditions occur. Consequently, diminishing one's positive outlook causes a person to sink into depression and lower his estimation of self-worth.

Physical activity is critical in achieving and maintaining wellness. Such helps to combat early mortality or sudden death syndrome. Physical activity will help to increase bone mass, strengthen the heart, shed pounds, regulate blood pressure, combat the effects of stress, and improve brain function and immune response. When the body aches, craves, diminishes, or is sick, it cries out for much-needed attention to help it get back to the purpose God intended. Again, this is how one attains wisdom regarding one's health. Too many are not listening to their bodies' cries for help as they settle themselves into the sedentary lifestyle of our time. Even children, who should be lively and full of energy and vitality, are succumbing to this fatal fact of a sedentary life. The phrase that most describes what happens to those who insist on remaining in such a lifestyle is "Sedentary Death Syndrome." Many will die because they did not take the steps necessary to promote health and wellness within themselves. In other words, for most people, it is within their power to determine how long they will live, how happy they can live, and how healthy they can live.

The secret to a full and happy life is not found in a pill, a fountain, or a machine. People want things now with minimal effort. There are drive-thru windows at food places and microwaves in every home. However, effort MUST be applied to achieve the life-sustaining goals necessary for health and wellness. Fredrick Douglass once said, "If there is no struggle, there is no progress." People want the results without effort. That is not how God made man.

Man must have physical activity in his life to be healthy and well. However, let us distinguish between physical activity and exercise. Physical activity encompasses any movement that contracts the muscles and raises metabolism. This would include mopping the floor, making a bed, washing dishes, etc. Exercise is a subcategory of physical activity geared toward achieving or maintaining physical fitness. It is usually of a higher intensity than regular physical activity. With the sedentary lifestyles of most today (we don't have to hunt, plant, plow, harvest, walk to work, etc.), low to moderate levels of exercise are necessary for anyone to continue to do effectively, the regular physical activities of everyday life. Whether with physical activity or exercise, the body's cells are jolted out of their resting state, followed by a complex energy production process to give the cells what they need to continue their course of activity.

With regular exercise, the benefits are tremendous. Improvements to a person's looks and the way they feel are only the tip of the iceberg in achieving wellness. One's health will improve, and one's life will be extended. He will also lower the risk of developing disabilities as he ages. Such activity reduces the chances of developing fatal illnesses like heart disease, diabetes, and cancer. If I can make a list of the expected benefits of regular moderate exercise, accompanied by good eating habits, this list would include:

- Weight control
- Better sleep
- Low risk of cancer
- Better mental health
- Increased flexibility
- Increase bone density
- Muscular strength, growth, and development
- Avoid early death
- Increase energy
- Overall wellness

Personal Training: Providing Optimal Health and Lifestyle Management

Personal Training is a highly structured, progressive, and practical lifestyle management system. It is ideal for preventing and relieving debilitating and degenerative conditions that would affect the body. The personal trainer's attention to functional movements and fitness progression allows anyone to participate in a training program. One of a personal trainer's fundamental functions is to promote optimal health. Everything that exercise and fitness experts suggest is necessary to combat and overcome a sedentary lifestyle and poor fitness habits; a quality personal trainer will do. The personal trainer will design fitness programs that will accommodate and be effective for everyone. The trainer will consider each client's age, fitness level, and health issues in developing their fitness program. The exercises will be tweaked along the way enabling clients to do well into their senior years. Such will increase vitality and longevity of life. Not only that, the time one spends on the earth will be healthy and productive years. Again, it is not enough to live long if you are not living well. Based upon pure science, when done correctly and regularly, personal training will help to make life worth living.

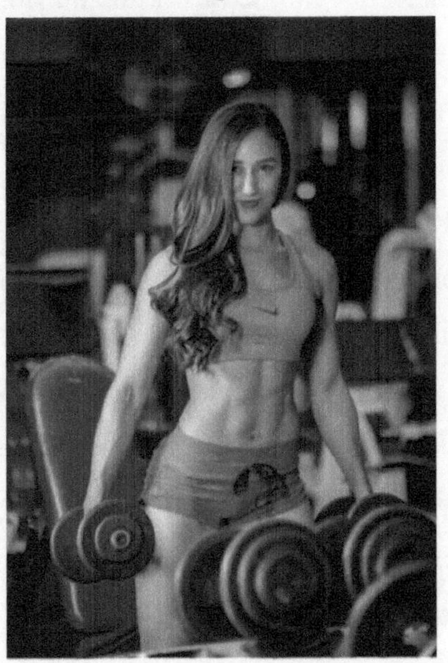

Personal Training and Health Clubs

We live in an age where physical fitness is a significant concern for most individuals. The Center for disease control cites that physical activity is vital for preventing chronic disease and promoting health. The American College of Sports Medicine and the American Medical Association teamed up to launch the "exercise is medicine" initiative. They believe that doctors should prescribe exercise to their patients. This is so people can make exercise a part of their daily routine. The American Cancer Society acknowledges and recommends exercise to aid cancer recovery and improve the quality of one's life. The evidence is overwhelming that exercise and physical fitness is necessary for a healthy and productive life. The question that must be asked is, "What kind of exercise program is ideal for optimal health benefits?"

It is incredible how many people believe that those who participate in athletic competitions are the epitome of health and fitness. Many want to aspire to be like these athletes. They fail to know that the intensity involved in training for athletic competition is detrimental in the long term. That is why professional athletes' careers are not long. In the NFL, the average career span is 3.5 years; NBA 4.8 years; MLB 5.6 years; NHL 5.5 years. Such has the opposite effect of moderate, regular exercise. Professional athletic training intensity increases free radical production, which is responsible for the breakdown of body function and the onset of aging. If a person is going to achieve optimal health and fitness, it is not enough just to exercise. His exercise regimen must be practical and proper, with the right intensity, frequency, and duration. Most people looking to get back into shape and physical fitness need guidance and instruction. This is where the certified personal trainer comes in.

Too many people believe that their hope for health and fitness lies in purchasing a health club membership. They psych themselves into believing that if they pay their money into a long-term contract with a health club, they will somehow be forced to deal with their fitness goals. But are gym memberships necessary and effective in achieving fitness goals and optimum health? With the expense, atmosphere, and activity involved with a gym membership, a mobile certified personal trainer will be a more effective, holistic, and even economical way to achieve optimal health and fitness.

The Pros and Cons of Health Club Memberships

Most people that sign on the dotted line for gym memberships believe that they are getting a bargain and that the gym has the remedy they need to attain physical fitness. Most health clubs that sign people up for membership are usually interested in getting the members' money and not in the members' fitness goals. Some of the downfalls of the gym membership that surveys have found are:

- **Time wasted waiting for machines to come available.** Not available machines perpetuate this because they do not work.

- **Filthy workout area.** Many of these clubs are generally not clean.

- **People who do not know how to use the machines.** Such leads to the machine break down and potential harm to the individual.

- **A lack of personal attention to attaining fitness goals from the staff.** Staff that is not adequately trained to handle the various fitness concerns that many have.

- **Lack of motivation**. Yet those that sign on the dotted line at a health club are always motivated to keep up their payments.

- **No praise for any strides in physical fitness the member may attain.**

- **The added expense for personal training.**
- **Boredom from hitting training plateaus.**
- **No guidance for proper training techniques.**

For some, going to a gym is motivation enough to avoid a sedentary lifestyle. Indeed, any reason for physical activity is a positive thing. Several gyms offer group fitness classes, which are certainly a better training method than going at it alone. More health clubs are turning to group fitness. Group fitness provides the support of others. However, there is usually one instructor in clubs and a class full of members. The instructor cannot care for everyone in the room. Fitness experts agree that the group fitness approach has been done successfully for years in martial art schools. As one who had previously worked at a gym as a fitness instructor, I can certainly attest to the pros and cons of going to a gym or health club. Most people who sign up for a health club membership become disenchanted with it after about 22 days. Anyone who becomes a member of a health club must contend with the machines on their own. The new member does not know how the machine works or what intensity they should train. I was in the gym, and I came upon a woman vomiting in a garbage can. I knew to ask her how long she had been coming to the gym. She was at the gym for the first time. As I began to advise her and aide her, a personal trainer from the club stepped in to take over. Now, I felt terrible for her. I do not know if that health club does a wellness profile. This woman may have had some impediments that needed to be addressed in her training.

A person, nonetheless, cannot get up and start training without a logical and practical approach to progression. A wellness profile that includes medical history, a physical activity readiness form, a waiver of liability, and a fitness assessment is necessary to provide a proper and effective fitness service. While many gyms and health clubs offer a variety of cardio and weight machines that a person can use along with a variety of fitness classes, the club member usually still does not know how to approach these things. To get the aid of an overpriced, underqualified personal trainer that these clubs have to offer is almost an insult. Even as an employee of a health club, I never would recommend a personal trainer for any of the members. Having observed them for quite some time, they were not adequately informed enough to provide an effective exercise program for those who would sign onto their program. Aside from the personal trainer, those who rely solely upon health clubs to achieve optimal health will quickly become discouraged. Unless the person who is a health club member is a seasoned athlete who knows the fundamentals of training, that person has many obstacles to overcome.

My observation as a fitness instructor at a health club grants me an insight others may not have. Those that rely upon fitness machines often plateau when they have been on them for a while. The machines do not fully accommodate the fitness level of the user. Indeed, they will achieve some level of fitness because of the exercise. However, the exercise machine reaches a maximum level that may not be as challenging as necessary. I used to do the recumbent bike at the maximum level for an hour and did not have the results I felt indicated the effort. I ran into the proverbial brick wall.

Unless a person switches up machines to challenge the body, he will run the risk of hitting a plateau in his fitness regimen. Many who go to health clubs or gyms repeatedly perform the same routines. Initially, there will be improved fitness and weight loss. However, over time, the body and muscles become more proficient in executing the movements associated with the exercise routine. Having adapted to the movements of the exercise routine, the muscles require less energy resulting in fewer calories burned. The exerciser falls into a fitness rut. He then becomes discouraged and eventually abandons his fitness regimen. Though most health clubs provide a variety of cardio and fitness machines, human beings are highly habitual, thriving on routines and rituals, making it easy for them to fall into a fitness rut in a health club environment. Because in most health clubs, the members are on their own and do not have the necessary motivation to overcome their fitness rut, in their despair, they quit.

The reason the rut happens is temporary. After a certain exercise period, the body goes into "under construction" mode. The body takes the time to build up its intracellular machinery necessary to meet its next fitness level. Fitness plateaus do not need to happen, however. With a proper diet and exercise program, a person can attain optimal fitness and avoid fitness ruts. My observation is that those who work out in health clubs tend to work out either at high intensity or insufficient intensity. Works outs that are too high in intensity causing the muscles to burn more sugars than fat, reducing energy levels before and after exercise. Workouts that are too low in intensity promote slowness in fat burning and do not effectively program the body to be fit and lean. Another element that contributes to the plateau effect is that some may not be exercising long enough. They have inadequate cardiovascular exercise duration. My observations at the health club confirm this fact. Many get on a cardio machine for 10 to 15 minutes and call it a day. They are simply wasting their time.

Also, the exerciser needs frequency in his routine to optimize physical conditioning. Adding days of working out will maximize the rate of conditioning. Three to six days should be the range for any fitness-minded person to extend their cardiovascular training. Any cardio workout must be accompanied by two days of resistance or strength training in the week. I have known people at the health club that refuses to do any weight training. This is especially true of some women that fear they would get too bulky or muscular. After 25, women tend to lose muscle at five pounds per decade. Unless a woman is purposely striving for that muscular look, regular weight training will not cause her to look like a bodybuilder. Muscular fitness is necessary for efficient fat metabolizing, strength, posture, and performance of anatomical movements. Such training needs to incorporate proper techniques to avoid injury and maximize time and effort efficiency.

Many health club members will not get the training necessary to maximize their health club experience unless they hire a personal trainer, dramatically increasing the cost of their health club membership. With the growing concern over health and fitness, how can anyone afford to invest in an effective program to allay such concerns?

The Benefits of Martial Art Training

Universal Martial Art is a highly effective and efficient martial art system. Its primary focus is self-defense. The practitioner will increase his confidence in his ability to thwart an attacker because of the effectiveness of the kicks and punches that make up Universal Martial Art. Universal Martial Art movements are very sophisticated. To perform the movements, the practitioner must focus on the complexity of the movements and the proper techniques.

The Universal Martial Art techniques are rooted in scientific principles. These principles include anatomy, physiology, kinesiology, psychology, and biomechanics. Biomechanics especially factor into the effectiveness of Universal Martial Art. Biomechanics concerns itself with the mechanics of movement involved with living organisms. When applied to human movement, the biomechanical principles incorporated in Universal Martial Art techniques help assure that those techniques are proper, safe, and effective. When combined, hand and foot techniques form Universal Martial Art patterns and speed drills. Each pattern and speed drill progresses in sophistication and complexity with each belt level in the Universal Martial Art system. This is because the sophistication and complexity of the kicks and punches in Universal Martial Art progress with each belt level. When students perform Universal Martial Art patterns and speed drills, they will progress in their fitness level with each new belt level. Universal Martial Art patterns and speed drills provide an adequate and effective aerobic exercise when students perform them at a moderate level of intensity. The large movements involved in performing the Universal Martial Art techniques provide the necessary stimulus for proper muscular development, which is a key to attaining optimal health.

Weight regulation, metabolic rate, and energy levels rely upon proper muscular function. Universal Martial Art takes into consideration the biomechanics of muscular function. The Universal Martial Art movements promote healthy slow-twitch function through the aerobic aspects of performing the patterns. Students can perform speed drills and bag work anaerobically, which helps to promote healthy fast-twitch muscular function. Bag work or target training also promotes lean muscle mass, increases bone density, and helps strengthen muscles. Because Universal Martial Art patterns and techniques progress with each belt level, students will always continue to challenge their cardio fitness levels. As each student progresses in Universal Martial Art, they add to their fitness program. Students learn a new hand technique, foot technique, pattern, and speed drill with each belt level. They can perform all the series of patterns and speed drills they learned with each new belt at one time, increasing the duration of their workout.

Because each Universal Martial Art instructor is certified and highly trained, each is capable of monitoring and assessing the production of every individual student. Since the students are a part of a class, they develop familial relationships, making their workout experience enjoyable. Universal Martial Art classes are available several days a week, making it possible for the student to train several days a week. The typical Universal Martial Art Class for adults lasts 45 minutes. The class begins with 10 minutes of dynamic stretching to warm up. Then the class performs basic techniques for 10 minutes. The class performs 10 minutes of patterns and 10 minutes of speed drills. The class concludes with five minutes of static stretching. This type of class is offered three days a week. The other three days replace the basic techniques, patterns, and speed drills with 15 minutes of defense drills and 15 minutes of target training. Six days of Martial Art training will provide an effective and proficient method of exercise that benefits every aspect of human health. Universal Martial Art classes offer the right level of intensity to meet the needs of everyone. The classes offer the recommended duration to attain cardiovascular health and provide an adequate frequency range.

The nine physical components of the Universal Martial Art system offer a complete body workout. Because Universal Martial Art is non-competitive, the participants have a fun, enjoyable, and non-stressful environment in which to train. Consider what a person would have to pay a health club to get close to that level and quality of training. Again, most people who attend health clubs do not know the proper way to train. So, they need to fork over hundreds of additional dollars for a personal trainer. A person will pay about $400 for six sessions with a personal trainer at most health clubs. This is on top of the $39 a month they were already paying to join that club. Most personal trainers have a one size fits all approach. Incorporating martial arts in personal training can cost as low as $299 a month for individual training and even cheaper in groups with no gym costs. As a personal trainer, I can even come to you. So, this eliminates the cost of travel.

Member-driven health clubs have a high turnover rate. One of the health and fitness clubs' dirty little secrets is that they oversell their memberships. They depend upon 80 to 90 percent of those who sign up not showing up to use the gym. And they don't care if the member honors his contract. If everyone who signed up came to the gym simultaneously, the fire marshal would have to close it down. Most of the people that go to these gyms look the same a year later. Universal Martial Art does not leave its members high and dry. They provide a clean school, a warm atmosphere, and a safe, non-competitive environment. Its instructors are highly trained, providing quality instruction. It is cost-effective. Those that sign up get their money's worth. Universal Martial Art offers excellent fitness benefits that help attain optimal health and even disease prevention when done correctly and regularly. With the support of instructors and fellow Universal Martial Art members, students receive recognition, encouragement, and motivation. Universal Martial Art provides 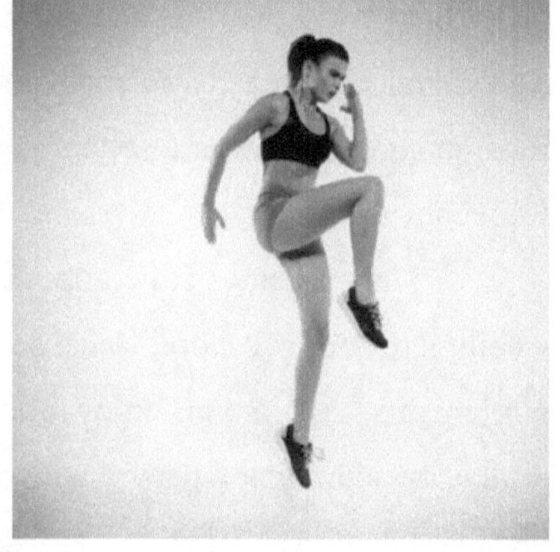 the students with every incentive to keep up with their training. The students come to a place they enjoy and from which they benefit.

The Brain and Personal Training for Children

A quality personal trainer will understand personal training that pertains to those of all ages and fitness types and how such movement will improve all aspects of the human body. One area of the human body that most never consider regarding personal training is the brain. There is a connection between movement in the form of exercise and brain development. Specific movement or exercise can affect the senses, emotions, speech, thinking, etc. Much of these elements are the products of the human brain. Without a properly developed brain, a person's sensory perceptions will diminish, his emotional well-being will suffer, and even such will affect one's speech. There are delicate intricacies of the brain. The brain connects other body systems to it in a way that helps the individual understand the importance of a well-tuned brain. Such affects the way a person breathes, the condition of a person's heart, proper organ functions, muscular and skeletal development, etc. When it comes to children, those who have time for structured play activities and regular exercise will have brains that will develop better than those who are more sedentary. Parents that do not allow their children to crawl may experience children that develop poor learning skills. The contralateral movement in the child's crawling helps to stimulate neural development, particularly in the brain.

Kids who play and exercise tend to be more successful in school. I remember that my grades were much better in school when I was active in sports. Even simply drinking the right amount of water a day helps to ensure proper brain development. The brain needs water to help protect it. The water provides a cushion to keep the brain bouncing off the cranium. In addition, water helps to ensure proper oxygen flow to the brain. The brain is a marvelous structure in that it will do what it must to survive. When a person starves himself, to help the brain survive, the body will metabolize muscle to bring energy to the brain. Proper exercise will go a long way to bring the brain what it needs to be healthy. Not only does the movement aid in learning and development, but it also helps the body to meet its demand for water and oxygen so that the brain will have what it needs to be healthy.

All should want to see children develop healthy minds and bodies as a society. To help our bodies, we must take care of our heads. We must have a greater appreciation for the brain. Most fail to realize what is necessary to keep it healthy. Most take their brains for granted. They do not appreciate how important the brain is in their overall health. I believe that children today face many learning disabilities simply because of inactivity. They are stressed, fat, irritable, and restless because they are inactive. School systems must dummy down academics because children cannot handle the challenges of learning at a higher level. Kids used to study Latin, Philosophy, Humanities, etc. Now kids can barely read. Schools have taken away physical education and recess where kids play. Even parents do not play with kids anymore. This has led to developmental problems in the brain, which results in poor learning skills.

Martial arts training can go a long way in helping develop a child's brain. However, not just any martial art will do. Because it is based upon scientific principles, Universal Martial Art will go a long way in ensuring the child practitioner's neurological development. Now, having that understanding, such will help me to be able to explain better the benefits of a Universal Martial Art program for students of any age. This goes a long way in explaining the distinction between Universal Martial Art training and training in traditional martial arts. When it comes to movement and exercise, it is not just an act of movement that matters, but the right kind of movement. Most traditional martial art systems use homo-lateral movement in their training. Such will hinder proper brain development.

Universal Martial Art training emphasizes optimal overall health. It is not enough to have healthy bodies; we need to have healthy brains. For children and adults, this type of development will improve production, and learning capacity, improve lives, and make an outstanding contribution to the health of any society. This is what Universal Martial Art in personal training is all about.

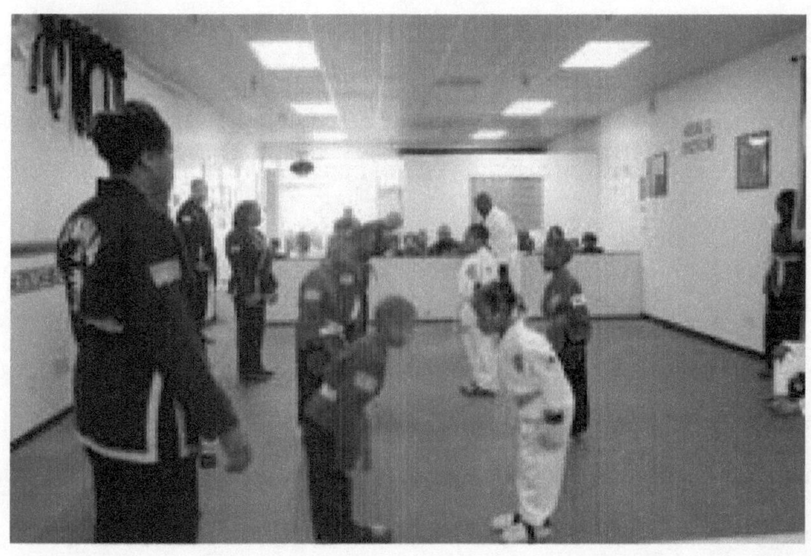

Personal Training and Seniors

God has designed the body to be and remain active, even into the golden years. Addressing these concerns early will slow down and even reverse the aging process so that a person can get back to a functional level that they once had in earlier years. For cardio health, flexibility, strength, and endurance to remain into the golden years, those at that age must remain physically active. Seniors can reap the benefits of weight management, disease prevention, mental fitness, better sex life, balance, agility, and longevity from continuous exercise. They must consider the quality of their exercise program and how overexertion from competitive training is counterproductive. I recommend low to moderate exercise for 45 minutes (at least) 6 days a week. Also, seniors should incorporate strength training two days each week. The exercise must be intense enough to make a difference.

I like to use the analogy of those who, in primitive times, had to hunt and farm for their food, to drive home the importance of physical activity. These activities demanded high levels of exertion. When they weren't hunting or farming, they danced and played active games. Even their diet was organic and very nutritious. They did not have to contend with preservatives or processed foods. Our ancestors were in tribes and had a tight familial relationship. This helped maintain happy and healthy relationships that aided in the prevention of mental stress and depression. It is no wonder that life expectancy at that time was very high (Gen. 5:1-32). Their genetic structure heeded the messages that stimulated growth, life, and happiness.

With a sedentary life and isolation, early death is inevitable. In code, we must speak to our body's most primitive instincts in a way it can understand, stay active, and connect. When we are sitting alone with a beer in hand in front of a TV, eating a processed snack and greasy foods, we tell our bodies to shut down and that our work on earth is done. We live in an age conducive to promoting a sedentary lifestyle. For that reason, the need to exercise is even more paramount. Seniors must embrace the mental attitude necessary for attaining a healthy lifestyle.

There is a need to establish relationships, to love and be loved. There is a need to serve our fellow man, our families, and ourselves. All of this shows a purpose for us to wake up every morning. We must establish the will to want to live long and healthy lives.

Seniors must focus on the need to eat healthily. Our eating habits must be good to best complement our pursuit of physical fitness. Some foods are beneficial, and others are detrimental to optimal health. In a word, I would like to call upon all of us to get back to what our ancestors were: athletes. For the greater part of human history, men and women challenged their bodies with activity. They were better able to combat disease and aging. Their bodies were "hard-wired" to do the tasks they needed to do each day. We don't have to hunt, farm, or walk in our age. We don't have to leave our couches (TV, Laptops, pizza delivery). If we stop moving, we shrivel up and die. Why does this happen when it is not necessary?

Personal Training and Universal Martial Art (UMA) for Seniors

The ten components of UMA, nine physical and one mental, are just what the doctor ordered. The components promote cardiovascular health and fitness in a non-stressful way. UMA is not a competitive sport but a life-altering, health-sustaining activity. Such also promotes strength and flexibility with target training and stretching. Students practice UMA in a class setting, which helps them establish a bond with other students that keeps them connected socially. The goal-setting in UMA provides the incentive necessary to keep one getting up every morning. Whether it is striving toward a new belt, becoming an instructor, or opening a school, at every level, UMA offers the challenge to the individual that keeps them coming back for more. Over time the student develops a never die attitude (Pil Seung) which will carry them through life.

UMA techniques provide a safe and easy approach to physical fitness for seniors. This is the reason I love the idea of incorporating UMA into my personal training programs. If the quality of life and longevity is a concern, personal training for seniors is the way to go. Taking a concern in getting back to the primitive instincts that gave man longevity and quality of life in the past, will help man to get back to the glory that God intended.

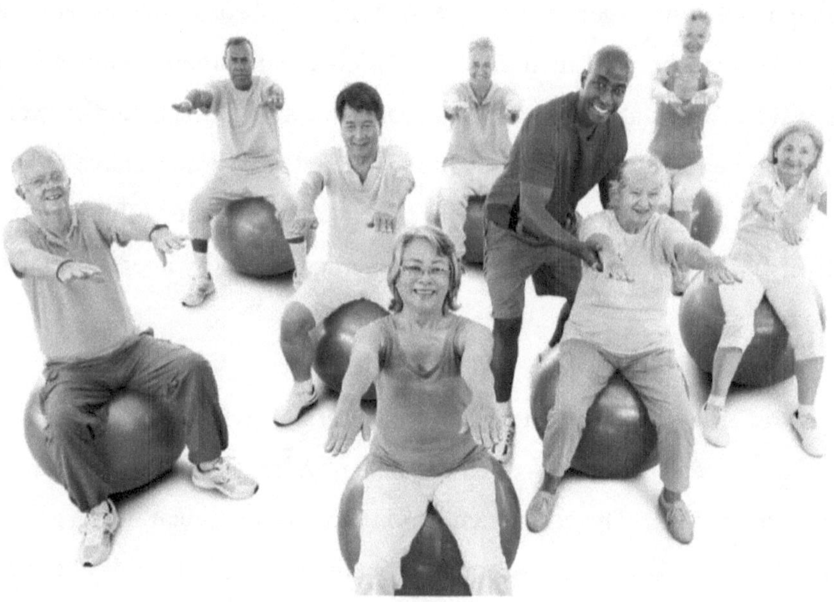

Personal Training and Stretching

Most people do not know the overall benefits of proper, consistent stretching. Most people associate stretching with trying to be more flexible. Some are reluctant to do it with any consistency because they feel that they cannot achieve the flexibility that many athletes have. This is possible because they are simply uninformed about the mechanics and benefits of stretching. There are many variations of stretching. Some are beneficial while others are not. Ballistic stretching, which once was thought to be beneficial, can lead to injury. This type of stretching uses the body's momentum to push the muscle beyond its normal range of motion. One would do this by bouncing into the stretch. This does not give the muscles a chance to relax into the stretch. Instead, the muscles would be prone to tighten because it activates the stretch reflex. Incorporated into the fundamentals of Universal Martial Art is a stretch routine. Based on years of study and analysis, Universal Martial Art utilizes proper fundamentals and techniques to ensure that the student obtains the maximum benefit from the stretch while at the same time lessening the risk of injury. Exercise should always strive to be a benefit, not a detriment to the overall health of the human body.

Why Stretch?

Today, so many lifestyles lend themselves to many of the health problems that they acquire. Sitting in front of computers and TVs and remaining sedentary has led to stiffness, aches, pains, and even joint problems. A person can prevent and overcome many of these ailments by simply taking time to stretch. It is essential to utilize our limbs' full range of motion and other moving body parts. The process by which the body achieves full range of motion (ROM) is through flexibility. ROM involves the movement around the joint or set of joints that connect to the ligaments, tendons, muscles, and bones. Many other factors affect flexibility: age, work activity, injury, etc. However, no matter the circumstance, with proper stretching, none of these factors should impede achieving good flexibility. Again, flexibility is necessary to achieve adequate performance in any physical endeavor. By maintaining good flexibility, a person can perform basic tasks such as walking correctly. Imagine how good and consistent Universal Martial Art stretching can help bolster a person's performance in more challenging physical activities.

What is Universal Martial Art Stretching?

Universal Martial Art stretching helps to lengthen the muscles, stimulate neural receptors, increase blood flow, relieve stress, and improve flexibility and overall performance. In Universal Martial Art, stretching is not a warm-up or something that is done simply as a precursor to doing Universal Martial Art but is an integral part of the Universal Martial Art System. Universal Martial Art stretching involves the following components: static stretch, dynamic stretch, and lower abdominal breathing.

A person performs the static stretch by elongating the muscle and holding it relaxed. The student should hold the stretch between 10 and 30 seconds. Holding the stretch for 30 seconds helps maximize the stretch's benefit. This type of stretch increases flexibility and provides vital nutrients and blood flow to the bones and joints. Bones are porous, allowing the elongated muscle squeezes blood to flow into the corresponding bone. Such helps to combat degenerative bone diseases such as Osteoporosis. The stretch can utilize another body part to hold it (passive). An example of this stretch would be the butterfly stretch that the student performs in Universal Martial (UMA). In addition, the student can perform the stretch by holding it without any assistance other than relying upon the strength of the agonist muscles (active). An example of this is the abdominal stretch that the student performs in UMA. The stretch also helps maintain good and proper posture, affecting the skeletal system.

A person performs the dynamic stretch by using controlled arm and leg swings that take the limbs gently to the limits of their range of motion. Some studies show that dynamic stretching is most beneficial before engaging in dynamic activity. The student should not perform this type of stretching to the point of fatigue. The benefit of such stretching is to increase motion and speed in the movement. When it is time to perform the athletic endeavor, the student can do so with ease and comfort. Again, one should not confuse this type of stretching with the old style of ballistic stretching, which uses bouncing motion to achieve a stretch beyond the normal range of motion.

The student should incorporate lower abdominal breathing (LAB) with all stretching. Deep LAB is beneficial because it helps bring needed oxygen to vital organs. It also helps to detoxify the organs of the body. LAB also promotes better digestion. Science calls this process peristalsis. Those who perform LAB accomplish this by raising the abdominal area into the diaphragm, causing a wave downward, which pushes and keeps the food down so that it may digest adequately. (LAB) also aids in the combat of diseases by triggering the lymphatic system, which is a vital agent in maintaining a strong immune system. In addition, LAB helps build stamina in disease-fighting and athletic activity.

Other Benefits of the UMA Stretch

As Universal Martial Art looks to promote optimal health, the Universal Martial Art stretches have a vital role in achieving that goal. A significant benefit of the stretch is to promote greater flexibility. With greater flexibility, the student will be able to perform their techniques more efficiently, utilizing greater power and speed. The muscles will be able to contract with greater ease. Added to this is the benefit of minor muscle soreness. The student will not be as prone to injuries when performing the Universal Martial Art techniques. The student will also have the benefit of leading a less stressful life. The relaxed static stretching, for example, helps aid in the release of endorphins from the pituitary gland into the spinal cord and brain through neurotransmitters. This is the body's natural way of combating pain. When released, endorphins give the body a sense of well-being. This also goes a long way toward tackling stress. Pain is stress-related. Pain can occur because of physical or emotional stress. With stress, the body opens itself up to physical maladies: disease, sickness, and heart problems. In conjunction, the stretch helps regulate the hypothalamus, which regulates organ-related activities, food intake, emotions, sleep patterns, and sex drive.

The Universal Martial Art stretch is vital in helping to maintain these body functions. The person who engages in proper Universal Martial Art stretching will maintain optimal health and achieve a sense of well-being that affects good mental health. They will maintain appropriate eating habits that will aid in maintaining proper weight. They will be more restful and energetic because they will sleep better. They will have more excellent mental stability and focus in their life. They will be more vibrant and feel more alive with a sense of youthful vigor. Who would not feel good about him or herself after achieving all those benefits? As I mentioned earlier, the Universal Martial Art Stretch affects proper digestion and the elimination of wastes from the body. It also involves breathing and heart rate. It helps slow breathing and lowers the heart rate, thus calming the body. Experts agree that this stretching process positively affects the parasympathetic nervous system. The sympathetic nervous system will dominate if a person does nothing to trigger the parasympathetic nervous system. This means more stress, panic, and nervousness, leading to increased health risks.

UMA Stretching and Personal Training

Utilizing the Universal Martial Art stretches in personal training will help those sessions be more effective in assisting clients to achieve their personal fitness goals. As a personal trainer, I will utilize Universal Martial Art stretches in the programs that I develop for my clients. This is one of the things that distinguish me as a personal trainer.

Indeed, anyone can see why the Universal Martial Art stretch is a pillar in the Universal Martial Art system. Universal Martial Art is designed for self-defense, but more importantly, it also helps achieve optimum health for the practitioner. Is it any wonder why the Universal Martial Art Stretch goes a long way toward achieving that goal?

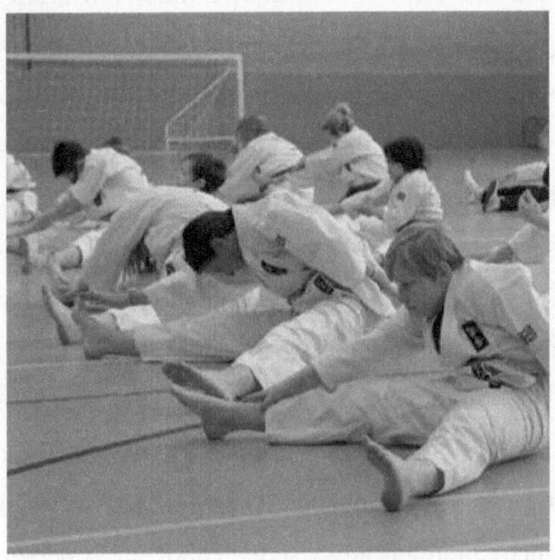

Personal Training and Resistance Training

Resistance training is a form of exercise that aids in muscle contraction against an outside force (resistance). These exercises can be isotonic (when the contracting muscle shortens against a constant load as when lifting a weight) or isometric (muscle contractions that occur without movement of the involved body parts; muscle fibers maintain a continuous length). Resistance training results in hypertrophy (an increase in the girth of the muscle). A person can lose cellular and organ size without such training.

Benefits of Resistance Training

Besides increasing muscle size and bone density, resistance training can help to contribute to improved performance in everyday activities. Isometric resistance training helps to develop the strength of an entire muscle group when one performs these exercises correctly. A person with arthritis can benefit tremendously from this form of resistance training. Arthritis involves the joints and is often aggravated when the person moves his joints. Isometric resistance training targets specific muscle groups around the joint without moving the joint. Isometric exercise strengthens the muscle groups putting less stress on the joints. The person will be better able to get around. Even with the aged, such training is essential because as a person ages, he loses about half a pound of muscle a year without such training. Strengthening the protagonist and antagonist muscles helps to keep the joints in their static position. Without such activity, a person compromises his ability to keep his balance. This is the reason falling is so prominent with the aged. Universal Martial Art is beneficial for people of all ages.

For this reason, it is dubbed "The Martial Art for everyone!" Another benefit to resistance training is increased metabolism. A person needs to consume more calories to maintain lean muscle mass. Muscles place a greater demand upon caloric absorption. Indeed, such is necessary for weight control. Some believe that aerobic exercise alone is enough to achieve optimal health. This is not so! While cardiovascular training may help build some muscle, it is not much. Muscles need to contract against resistance to maintain size, bone density, strength, and endurance. I mentioned the benefits of isometric training. However, such is limited because it does not adequately prepare one for more dynamic activity. Isotonic exercise (push-ups, sit-ups, leg raises, etc.) does this. While moving one's joints, one strengthens the surrounding muscles while at the same time conditioning the muscles to perform in coordination with the full range of motion of the isotonic exercise. Other benefits include improved blood pressure, balance, absorb shock, improved body composition (tone), and a lower risk of injury. A person will be able to perform everyday tasks with less effort and for a longer duration. Muscles will ultimately improve their capacity to perform.

Resistance Training and Universal Martial Art

When we condition our muscles properly for strength, size, and endurance, this will help us in our ability to perform our Universal Martial Art techniques better. Without resistance training, much of what we do in Universal Martial Art helps to improve mainly our aerobic and anaerobic capacity. Resistance training helps with our power, speed, and

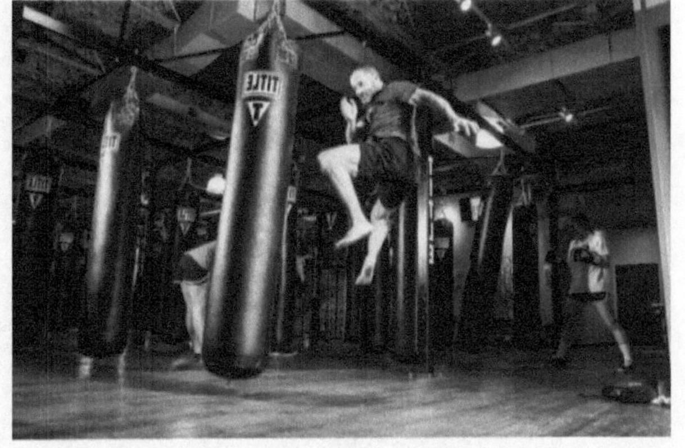

accuracy as we perform Universal Martial Art techniques. The foresight and genius to incorporate resistance training in Universal Martial Art offer more evidence to suggest that Universal Martial Art stands alone in the Martial Arts world. No one else has these fundamental components in their martial art. Universal Martial Art is a leader in providing the necessary tools to achieve optimum health. A practitioner derives greater flexibility when one reaches a full range of motion through Universal Martial Art stretching. He derives cardiovascular fitness from aerobic and endurance training in Universal Martial Art. The practitioner will achieve this fitness level by performing Universal Martial Art techniques, patterns, speed drills, defense drills, and close-range attacks. He derives strength through resistance training. This helps increase the Universal Martial Art student's ability to perform at his level best. By attaining the goals set out in Universal Martial Art's flexibility, cardiovascular, and resistance training, the practitioner will achieve optimal health and prevent debilitating, degenerative conditions that afflict many people today.

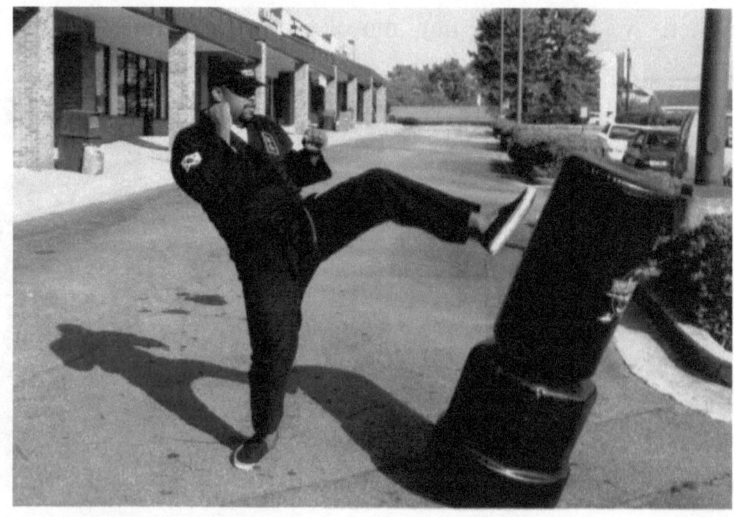

Applied Science in Personal Training

Applied science is the exact science of taking knowledge from one or more fields of natural science and using it to solve practical problems. We take the years of learning from the various fields of science and incorporate them into Universal Martial Art. By performing the Universal Martial Art techniques, a person can prevent and combat many health problems they face daily. Most of the health problems that plague society today are the consequences of specific human behaviors. In other words, many diseases and illnesses people have brought upon themselves. Obesity, for example, having too much body fat (differs from being merely over-weight – muscle weighs more than fat), is a condition that is a direct result of poor eating habits or a lack of exercise, or both. This means that it is within the purview of every individual to control this problem. While many may not consider obesity a disease, such puts a person at risk for disease or health problems (diabetes, high blood pressure, heart disease, stroke, arthritis, and even some cancers).

Now let us consider how we can utilize applied science concerning this problem of obesity. Scientific studies have shown that the human genetic structure was programmed some 10,000 years ago to anticipate physical exertion. God designed the human genome to function within the extensive physical activity. Before the dawning of the age of technology, humanity had to hunt for food, work the fields, travel by foot most of the time, etc. He did not have the opportunity or time for many sedentary activities. He had no computers, no TVs, phones, or PlayStations. He had to utilize the daylight time to get his work done. Because they had no electricity, when dusk came upon men, they went to sleep for the night (regenerating from the daytime activities).

Interestingly, men lived longer than they do today, about 10,000 years ago, especially during the antediluvian period. They engaged in physical activity, ate organic foods (grains, fruits, and vegetables), and ate very little red meat. Now move to our time. We get our food and eat our food without even leaving the seat of our cars, never mind the kind of food that we are eating. Because of technology, people today do not seem to have much reason to be active. Scientific research has shown that this dramatic lifestyle change altered our genetic makeup over time. Because of the lack of physical activity, compounded with the type of diets most have today, has altered the protein expression of cells today, leading to cellular breakdown and chronic health disorders. Even when those in ages past were not hunting, toolmaking, farming, etc., they did engage in other forms of physical activity. A study of past civilizations uncovered that many of those cultures spent their downtime dancing. For a long time, dance was a part of everyday culture. Now, machines gather, cook, and even give us our food. Machines play our sports and games, and we watch people dance as we sit and drink our beers and eat our wings.

Without going back to the Stone Age, we can apply the knowledge we have learned from scientific research to solve today's health problems. Many had once believed that disease and other health disorders resulted from heredity. A person's bloodline predisposed his genes to break down and fail. I do not believe this to be true. I believe we have a genetic predisposition to be healthy. Our habits, environment, and even our social interactions play an essential part in determining our genetic outcomes. While it is true that our genetic structure has predetermined traits (hair color, eye color, height, lefty or righty), I do not believe that a person is predisposed to chronic disorders. Since man has gone through environmental, physical activity, nutritional, and even psychological changes over human existence, some believe this has altered how genes function and cellular fate. Science has termed this process Epigenetics. If a person can manipulate or influence genes in a way that adversely affects his health, why not manipulate those genes to affect his health favorably?

Since our age has evolved to make the intended use of the human genome obsolete, we must compensate for this for our survival. To maintain overall health, our intended genetic structure necessitates a certain level of physical activity. Now, to achieve this, we must exercise. Our exercise must have all the essential components necessary to achieve optimal health. Frequency, intensity, and duration are those aspects that an instructor or trainer can carefully help balance. Exercise must contain elements that help build endurance, strength, cardiovascular output, and flexibility. Sedentary lifestyles adversely affect muscular, skeletal, and nervous systems, leading to chronic, degenerative disorders.

Universal Martial Art and Applied Science

Universal Martial Art goes a long way in helping to achieve these fitness goals by utilizing applied science principles. Universal Martial Art rests upon ten pillars that make up the system.

These pillars are:
1. Warm-up and Cool-down
2. Stretching
3. Basic Techniques
4. Patterns
5. Speed Drills

6. Defense Drills

7. Close range Attack Drills

8. Target Training

9. Resistance/Strength Training

10. Character Development

Anyone who consistently practices Universal Martial Art will be able to defend oneself and combat degenerative conditions in the body. The body will adapt to our demands and thus prepare it to meet those demands. With physical exertion, the body tends to prepare itself to meet the demands of that type of activity. This is like a person that tries to lose weight by starving himself. The body adapts by storing calories and slowing metabolism. Our genetic make-up lives for exertion. The exertion produces the protein expression within the genes necessary to survive. Without physical exertion, we will die. A person lying in a hospital bed immobile will atrophy and develop sores. Bedsores develop because there is no movement in those areas, and the skin dries and breaks down. This, combined with the continuous pressure placed upon that area, decreasing blood flow, makes for an unpleasant situation. Just imagine what would become of the person who has no physical activity.

Universal Martial Art provides energy and enhances circulatory activity during the warm-up, cool-down, and stretching. Combined with proper lower abdominal breathing, such will bolster our disease-fighting capabilities. Performing the basic techniques and patterns in Universal Martial Art helps to stimulate our cellular development and achieve our predetermined genetic purpose. The speed, defense, and close-range drills will help build our stamina and increase our aerobic capacity. Target training will help improve our coordination and strength by stimulating our muscles, tendons, and bones. Resistance training will improve muscle growth, strength, and neuromuscular efficiency. Character development also helps to improve the quality of our health and life. When we are happy and secure, our stress levels are down, and even our free radical production diminishes. Anger, hostility, depression, and anxiety influence a person's health. Universal Martial Art principles help to guide a person toward a more controlled mental environment and happy existence. Loving relationships and peaceful environments all have a place in improving the quality of a person's health and life.

You cannot find this quality and well-rounded type of physical exercise anywhere else. Competitive sports are ego-driven, thus adding to increased stress and anxiety to perform. The exertion needed to perform at such levels of competition is detrimental to the body and often has the opposite effect that most hope exercise would achieve. Even the gym or health club cannot provide such an overall health benefit because it does not engage the mind. Other martial arts do not have the components necessary to address the needs of the 21st century concerning human health and development. That is why Universal Martial Art is the martial art for the 21st Century and the martial art for life.

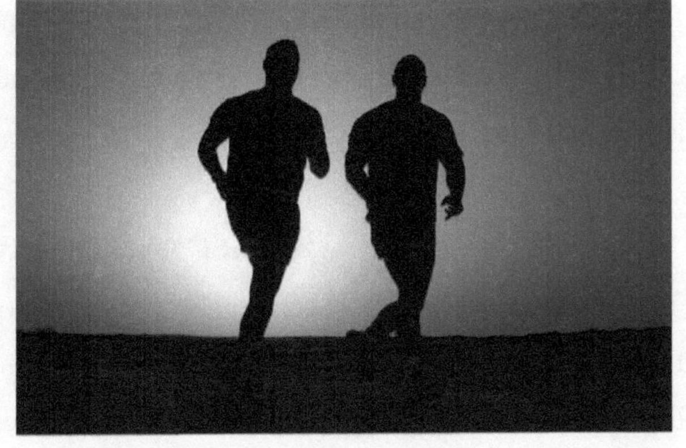

Personal Training and Obesity

Obesity occurs when a person accumulates body fat over 20% of his ideal weight. Health experts associate obesity with an increase in illness, disability, and even death. The higher the body fat percentage over the ideal weight, the more one increases the risk of adverse effects. A more recent method of determining obesity is measuring Body Mass Index (BMI). To calculate BMI, a person must multiply his weight by 703 and divide it by height in inches twice. BMI over 30 is obese. Obesity strains the organs and joints and often leads to degenerative diseases such as type II diabetes, hypertension, heart disease, and even certain cancers. The World Health Organization has deemed obesity a worldwide epidemic and has noted the diseases associated with obesity to be more prevalent. Recently the WHO has linked obesity to six different types of cancers. Obesity, therefore, is not simply an appearance issue but also affects a person's health in the manner previously mentioned. It also affects the quality of a person's life. Obesity affects energy levels, sleep, mood, and even breathing. This is a problem for more than just adults. One-third of kids between the ages of 2 and 19 are overweight or obese. Even at these young ages, kids show signs of degenerative health problems.

What Causes Obesity

A variety of factors can combine to trigger obesity. For some, it is genetic. For others, it is the environment. For most, it is simply a matter of behavior and lifestyle. It seems reasonable to assume that our creator did not design the human body to carry excess fat. The body reacts negatively to anything detrimental to it. People are making unhealthy food choices. Eating fast, processed foods is not wise. Eating in front of a TV rather than around a dinner table can lead to obesity because a person cannot fully concentrate on eating. Eating larger portions and second helpings have become the norm. Eating when one is depressed, stressed, anxious or bored is a bad habit that often leads to obesity. Combine these behaviors with a sedentary lifestyle with little to no exercise, and you have a recipe for a health disaster.

Exercise and Obesity

Eating more calories than one burns causes those unused calories to be stored as fat. Usually, as a person gains weight and reduces physical activity, obesity will result. Some people believe that simply cutting calories is enough to conquer this epidemic. Ninety-Five percent of people, who lose weight in this manner, put the weight back on again. A person needs to tackle obesity with healthier food choices, eating habits, and exercise. The person who exercises will have improved fat loss. This fat loss will be for the long term for those who exercise instead of those who diet only. Those who exercise regularly and with a moderate level of intensity 5-7 days a week, accompanied by healthy eating habits, will do more for their health and obesity prevention than those who only cut calories. Consider some of the benefits of exercise: improved blood sugar control, lower LDL, lean muscle mass (which leads to increased energy and metabolism), lower blood pressure, and reduced risk of heart disease.

Universal Martial Art and Obesity

While exercise is essential in combating obesity, not all forms of exercise are conducive to helping meet the long-term goal of combating obesity. Some exercise programs are brutal and harsh and will soon discourage the practitioner because of the pain, soreness, and boredom accompanying such exercise. While a martial art designed for self-defense purposes, Universal Martial Art provides an excellent exercise for the practitioner. Universal Martial Art techniques and movements are not stress-related or too intense for the practitioner. The instructors deliver instruction in a non-competitive environment that makes the classes more exciting and pleasurable. The student comes to class with a goal-setting mindset. The student pledges, "To set positive goals and strive to achieve them." With each new belt level, the student challenges and heightens their fitness level. In addition, the student sets and strives for a new goal: the next belt. The benefits of performing Universal Martial Art in a class setting are tremendous. Studies have shown that those who exercise with other members are more successful in achieving their goals than those who exercise and diet alone. Universal Martial Art helps provide the physical activity necessary to combat obesity and helps to alter one's mental state concerning their image. Principals such as self-control, perseverance, and unbreakable spirit are crucial in instilling determination into the one trying to combat issues such as obesity. Since these goals are long-term, the student can perform Universal Martial Art for sustained periods. Also, because of the larger moments of both hands and feet, Universal Martial Art is more effective in fighting obesity and maintaining weight than

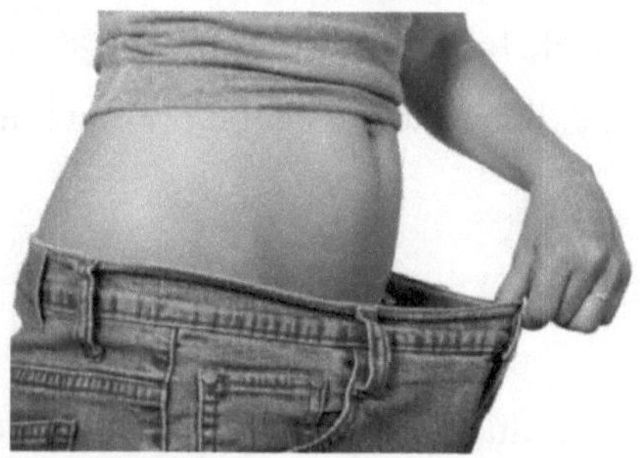

walking, running, or using any fitness machine. Whereas you cannot take your fitness machine anywhere you go, the student can perform Universal Martial Art anywhere, anytime, and in any environment. Universal Martial Art is ideal for combating obesity because it is always practical and available.

Personal Training and Cardiovascular Disease

Cardiovascular disease involves dysfunctions of the heart, veins, or arteries. These are responsible for bringing oxygen and nutrients to organs and tissue. If oxygen does not get to these vital body elements, they will die. Several ailments fall under the category of cardiovascular disease. To name a few, there are strokes, heart attacks, high blood pressure, and angina. Strokes are the result of poor oxygen flow to the brain. Heart attacks result from a blockage in one or more coronary arteries. This blockage is called plaque. Such denies oxygen-rich blood from reaching the heart muscle resulting in cellular destruction, and if a big enough area is damaged, it can cause instant death. Angina is chest pain that comes from the narrowing of the arteries. Angina can lead to heart attacks. High blood pressure is another major complication of cardiovascular disease. Blood pressure is necessary for the body to function properly. The force of the blood being pumped meets the resistance of the arteries in which the blood flows. In a healthy body, the arteries are elastic and stretch to adjust to the force of blood being pumped through them. Under normal conditions, your heart beats 60 to 80 beats per minute. Blood pressure should be less than 120/80 (millimeters of mercury). 140/90 suggests hypertension (high blood pressure). The higher number represents the systolic pressure (when the heart is pumping); the lower number represents the diastolic (when the heart is resting between beats). When you have high blood pressure, the force against your artery walls is too strong. Such can damage your arteries, kidneys, and heart. This often leads to stroke. High blood pressure is known as a silent killer in that, undetected, it can kill you without any symptoms.

Let us consider some of the causes of cardiovascular disease. Obesity, stress, sedentary lifestyle, salt intake, and alcohol intake are the major causes of cardiovascular disease. Such stands to reason that the major causes of cardiovascular disease are preventable. The prevention of such a debilitating disease incorporates a healthy diet and exercise. Many of the cardiovascular problems that occur directly result from sedentary lifestyles. According to a 2012 study, about 47% of Americans had cardiovascular disease (Fryar et al., 2012). As more people take charge of their lives and health, cardiovascular disease will diminish, and people will also have stronger hearts. Cardiovascular disease is one of those problems for which people can take responsibility. What a person does and eats has much to do with whether they will acquire this disease.

Exercise and Cardiovascular disease

Three reviews of over 50 observational studies have shown that the risk of cardiovascular disease was lower in physically active persons. The more inactive the person was, the greater his risk for cardiovascular disease. In many cases, this risk even doubled. A person needs to achieve moderate level exercise to benefit from the exercise. The person needs to exercise 150 minutes a week of moderate-intensity exercise or 73 minutes of high-intensity exercise. Beneficial cardiovascular exercise must consist of three vital components: duration, intensity, and frequency. Frequency is the most critical factor. A person should exercise at least three days out of the week. The next most important is duration. Each session must be between 30 and 45 minutes. The duration can be broken up into intervals.

Finally, based on cardiovascular fitness, the intensity must be at a pace that will help to increase heart and lung capacity. One can measure the VT1 and VT2 talk tests with this pace or intensity. At VT1 lactic acid begins to accumulate in the blood, making talking difficult. VT is the anaerobic threshold where talking is uncomfortable. At VO2 max, exercise must end as the participant will be out of breath. Most Americans do not participate in enough physical activity to acquire health benefits. The more exercise a person does, the more he lowers his risk of cardiovascular problems. The question is, how does exercise help to lessen the risk of cardio problems? While exercise does not directly reduce Cholesterol, it does help elevate HDL that counters LDL levels in the blood. Regular exercise along with a proper diet helps to combat obesity. People who increase their physical activity are less likely to smoke. Exercise helps the body metabolize carbohydrates more efficiently. As a person exercises, they help in the production of fibrinolytic activity. This activity keeps blood clots from forming by dissolving them. Exercise helps reduce high blood pressure and will help slow its rise when a person begins to age. With exercise, there is less demand for oxygen in the heart.

Universal Martial Art and Cardiovascular Disease

Most people do not sustain a cardiovascular exercise routine due to boredom and repetitiveness. Universal Martial Art is anything but dull. It offers an exciting and pleasurable exercise designed to stimulate the participant progressively. Universal Martial Art provides an exciting cardio exercise system with the constant challenge of learning new techniques, patterns, and speed drills. With the continuous use of hands and feet in performing Universal Martial Art, the cardiovascular system is opened faster and more efficiently than traditional exercise alone. The practitioners will have a stress-less environment with camaraderie and class structure. Exhibiting positive emotions can have tremendous benefits in aiding optimal health in as much as stress is bad for the heart. When the person is in a positive, encouraging environment like a Universal Martial Art class, such raises a joyous disposition in the person rather than the discouragement and disappointment of competitive athletics. A passage in the Bible summarizes this well, *"A merry heart does good, like medicine, but a broken spirit dries the bones"* (Pro. 17:22). Professional Universal Martial Art Schools are more than capable of meeting the needs of those looking to prevent cardiovascular problems. They provide the frequency with classes available several days each week. They provide duration as classes are at least 45 minutes each session. They provide intensity with patterns and speed drills that the students perform aerobically for health purposes.

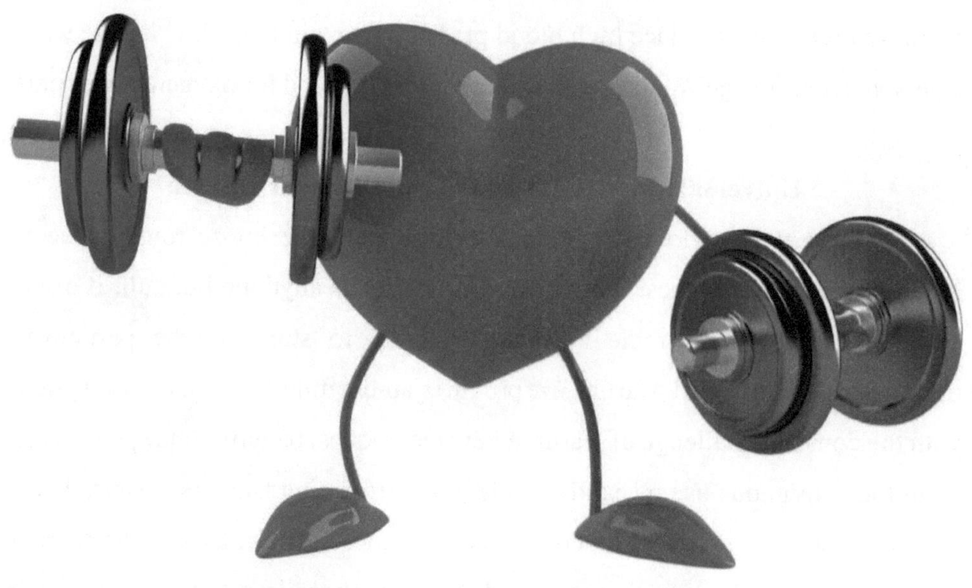

Personal Training and Diabetes

Scientists today believe that diabetes is not a single disease but a group of disorders that relate to abnormal glucose metabolism. Simply, diabetes is the body's inability to use the energy adequately from the food that it takes in. A person without diabetes can eat his food normally. The food breaks down into glucose. The glucose is then absorbed into the bloodstream, causing the blood glucose levels to rise. This sends a signal to the pancreas to produce and release insulin. Insulin is a hormone that causes glucose to move out of the bloodstream into the body cells. Here, glucose serves as energy for the body. When glucose moves into the cells, blood glucose levels fall. When a person has diabetes, the pancreas does not produce enough insulin, or the insulin it produces does not work correctly.

Several different types of diabetes produce the same result: high blood glucose levels.

Type I Diabetes Mellitus – This is the insulin-dependent type of diabetes. It occurs when the autoimmune system in the body begins to destroy the beta cells in the pancreas, causing it no longer to produce insulin. A person with type I diabetes must take insulin shots to survive. This type of diabetes usually occurs in childhood.

Type II Diabetes Mellitus – The person with type II diabetes has a relative insulin deficiency. This person may have either normal or excessive insulin levels in the bloodstream. Usually, the disorder results from the cell's inability to use insulin properly. Science regards this as insulin resistance. This type of diabetes is most common. Approximately 90% of all diabetes cases are type II. The person most likely to fit the condition is overweight, over 40 years old, and has a history of diabetes in the family. Symptoms usually come over a long period. The symptoms include:

- Fatigue
- Frequent urination
- Increased hunger and thirst
- Slow healing cuts
- Dry, itchy skin
- Blurred vision
- Numbness or tingling in hands or feet

Treatments that an expert prescribes for type two diabetes help enhance a person's ability to use his insulin better. Such treatments would include weight loss, a proper diet, regular exercise, and blood glucose monitoring.

Exercise and Diabetes

Exercise for the person with diabetes helps control and even lose weight, regulate blood sugar levels, and lower the risk of heart disease, common in people with diabetes. In addition, exercise helps to give a person a sense of well-being and improve overall health. Exercise changes the way the body reacts to insulin by making it more sensitive to insulin. Because most people with type II diabetes are overweight and have high cholesterol and high blood pressure, exercise is ideal to remedy the symptoms of diabetes and even prevent the onset of diabetes. Obesity is the number one risk factor for type II diabetes. More important than even diet to control obesity is moderate, regular exercise. Exercise helps regulate blood flow, increase metabolism, control weight, and improve cardiovascular performance. Exercise also lowers bad cholesterol while raising good cholesterol.

The other added benefits of exercise in treating type II diabetes are reduced stress and tension, relaxation, increased energy, and work capacity.

However, the exercise routine must be at the right level of intensity. When exercise becomes too strenuous or intense, the body treats such as added stress and could have the opposite effect on type II diabetes than originally intended. When a person incorporates strength training into the exercise program, such has a profound impact on blood sugar levels in the body. The body loses fat, utilizes insulin more efficiently, lowers cholesterol levels, increases a sense of well-being, and increases energy levels. The effect that strength training has in treating diabetes is comparable to, if not exceeds, treatment-using medicines.

Universal Martial Art and Diabetes

Medical experts agree that no treatment or prevention of type II diabetes can eliminate exercise. Universal Martial Art provides all the necessary components to aid in preventing and treating type II diabetes adequately. The Universal Martial Art patterns allow the practitioner to perform them aerobically at a moderate level of intensity. When the practitioner does this for five days, he will receive the exercise's benefits from 45-60 minutes each day. Combined with the resistance training from target training, practitioners will arm themselves with everything they need to combat this debilitating condition. A student who trains regularly in Universal Martial Art and eats right will have one less degenerative disease to worry about as they achieve optimal health. Personally, my endocrinologist diagnosed me with Type II diabetes back in 2006. Since then, using

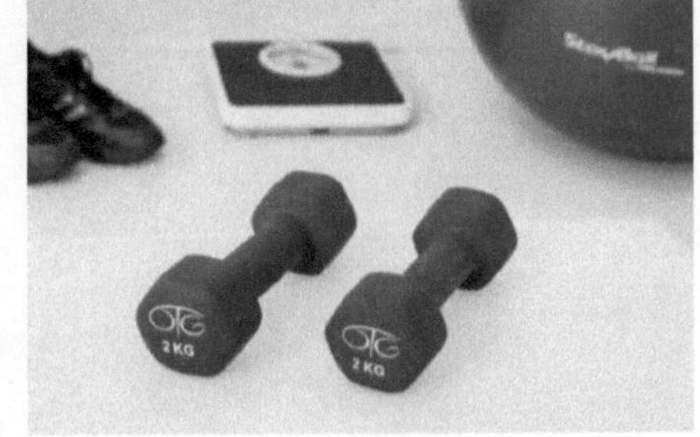

the tools I had at my disposal, Universal Martial Art, I began training at least five days a week for 1 ½ hour each day. With healthy eating, I lost 30 pounds and never experienced the symptoms of diabetes. My blood sugar averaged 93, staying between 80 and 120. Even the endocrinologist's nurses wondered why I was even a patient. I was 280 pounds in 2006. Now I am a fit 205 pounds without any diabetic symptoms.

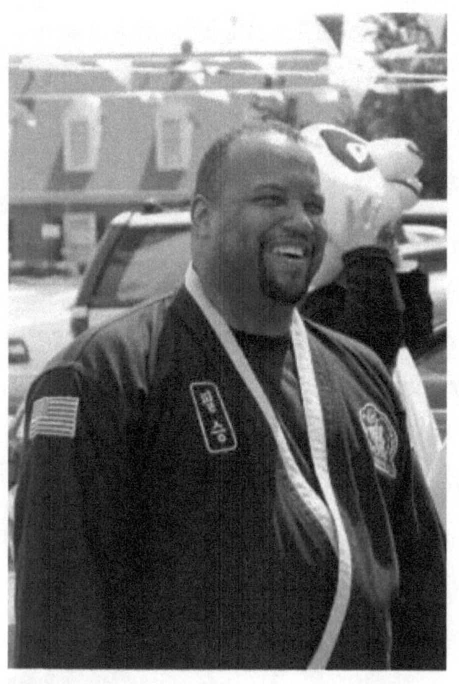
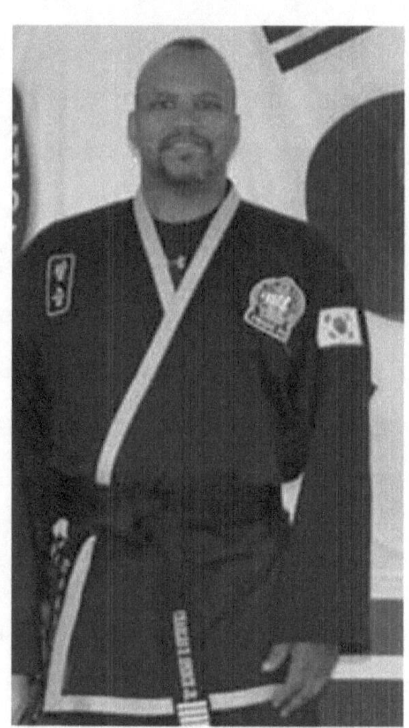

Personal Training and Cancer

Cancer is a disease characterized by abnormal growth of cells resulting in malignancy or carcinoma. There are over 100 different variations of cancer. The most common types of cancer are breast, skin, lung, prostate, and colon. Cancer develops when cells grow aggressively, dividing without respect to normal functions, invade and attack surrounding tissue, metastasize, and spread to other body parts. These three characteristics distinguish malignancy in tumors from benign. Cancer can affect anyone at any age; however, the more common cancer risks occur as people get older. About 13% of all deaths are cancer-related. Normal body function dictates that cells die and new cells grow. When cells grow faster than old cells die, tumors form. These tumors can either be malignant or benign, as discussed earlier.

Many types of cancer are caused by the things people do. Smoking leads to cancer of the mouth, throat, lungs, kidneys, bladder, and possibly other organs. Drinking too much alcohol can trigger cancer in the throat and mouth. A person who drinks and smokes multiplies the risk of cancer. All kinds of carcinogens (cancer-causing agents) factor into a person's life. Many cancer risks are preventable. Many health experts have linked obesity and physical inactivity to cancer risk. Obesity increases cancer risk in the breast, uterus, colon, kidney, and esophagus. Obesity and physical inactivity may account for 25 to 30 percent of significant types of cancer cases. In 2002 there were 41000 new cases of cancer estimated to be linked to obesity. Thus, such resulted in a 3.2 increase in cancer due to obesity. Fourteen percent of cancer deaths in men and 20 percent of cancer deaths in women were related to obesity. A conscientious person living a healthy lifestyle comprising of a healthy diet, avoiding harmful habits, and regular moderate level exercise will go a long way in helping to lower the risk of cancer growth. Most people live their lives with a blatant disregard for the risks and consequences of their chosen lifestyle. People overeat the wrong things and exercise too little; whether people realize it, sedentary lifestyles are killing them.

Exercise and Cancer

Studies have shown that physical exercise helps to reduce the risk of cancer. Physical exercise helps to improve overall health. Exercise helps to regulate the processing of energy. Regular, moderate exercise helps to reduce fat and combat obesity. Studies have shown that regular exercise helps to combat colon and breast cancer. Women athletes who continued their exercise had lower incidents of cancer than non-athletic women. Young girls who exercise regularly have shown lower risk incidents of breast and cancer of the uterus. Exercise has a tremendous effect on the immune system. A healthy immune system is vital for fighting destructive invasions of the body. However, the exercise must be moderate. Those who constantly work out at high-intensity levels and engage in athletic competitions increase their cancer risk. High-intensity exercise increases free radicals that alter and destroy the normal function of cells. However, this is temporary and will ultimately result in building oxidative resistance. Studies have also shown that exercise that does not have the right level of intensity provides no benefit in fighting cancer. For those with cancer, low to moderate exercise is beneficial for helping to provide energy and endurance during times of chemotherapy. Also, exercise is beneficial for combating the loss of strength and even bone density that comes with chemotherapy. Overall well-being and quality of life can be had for the person with cancer.

Universal Martial Art and Cancer

Universal Martial Art offers the practitioner a complete exercise routine. Universal Martial Art Schools provide several classes that allow the practitioner to train regularly. Universal Martial Art instructors are professionally trained and can guide the student in the right level of intensity to get the most out of the exercise. Moderate exercise helps alleviate stress and the production of free radicals in the body. Free radicals aid in cell damage. Universal Martial Art classes are carefully managed and monitored to provide the most significant benefit. Stretching, basic techniques, patterns, speed drills, defense drills, and target training combine to give the practitioner all the tools necessary to be fit. Universal Martial Art classes provide aerobic and anaerobic activities that provide the required intensity to the exercise. Universal Martial Art is an effective self-defense tool in combat situations; it also aids in defense against such debilitating diseases as cancer. Consistent training in Universal Martial Art with a healthy diet is everything a person needs to assist in the prevention of the major types of cancer.

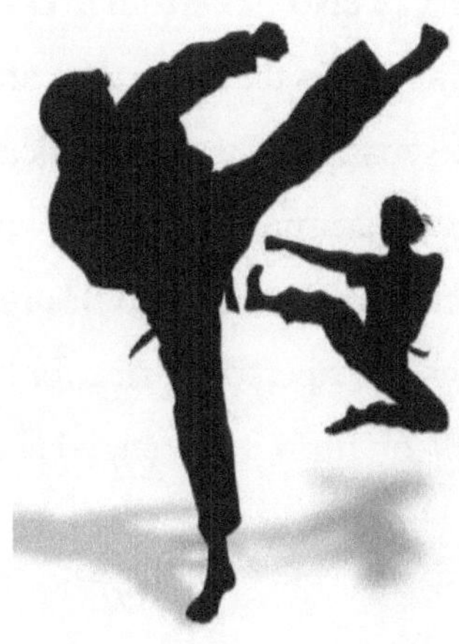

Personal training and Back Pain

Back pain affects 80% of people at some point in their lives. Annually 15 to 45% of people suffer from back pain. It is the most common reason people go to the doctor and miss work. 40% of workman's compensation goes to back pain sufferers. Back pain costs the industry billions of dollars in lost person-hours. In 1990 back pain cost American industry between 50 and 100 billion dollars. The annual health care cost for back pain is 20 to 50 billion dollars. Usually, back pain is a symptom of an underlying problem. Back pain can come in several forms: lower back, neck, and sciatica. To best treat back pain, one must determine its cause. Some controversy has arisen concerning the actual cause of back pain. Some have argued whether back pain results from trauma or is merely a condition likened to a headache. One thing is sure, outside of unavoidable trauma, back pain is preventable. The back is composed of disks, muscles, tendons, and ligaments that work intricately together. Back pain can stem from problems with any components that make up and support the spine. That is why it is hard to isolate the causes. Most back pains are associated with strains due to heavy lifting or sudden movement. Back pain can also stem from irregularities in the spine. These irregularities are ruptured disks (disks that over time are out of line because of the erosion of the cushion that separates them); sciatica (when a bulging disk is pressing upon the main nerve that runs up and down the leg); osteoporosis (a condition that leaves the bones weak and brittle); arthritis (affects the joints in hips and spine). Certain things put a person at risk for back pain. Those things are obesity, age, strenuous work or lifting, anxiety, lack of exercise or moderate physical activity, and stress. From what we can see, the risks to back pain are preventable.

Exercise and Back Pain

There is a great misconception about whether those who experience back pain should take it easy. Some health experts even suggest that a person with back pain commit to bed rest for days at a time. While Bedrest may be what one needs in the short term, such is detrimental in the long term. Studies and even experience have shown that such an approach can harm spinal healing. Moderate levels of exercise are almost always instrumental in promoting healing to the spine and alleviating back pain. Moderate exercise, when done properly, helps to distribute nutrients into the spaces between the disks, keeping the cushion soft and healthy. In addition, the muscles and ligaments that support the back are kept healthy. Regular exercise will help to prevent stiffness while strengthening the back. Also, such will go a long way to minimize the risks to back pain (obesity, stress, anxiety, etc.). Moderate exercise will also reduce the occurrences of back pain and reduce the severity and duration of future occurrences.

Universal Martial Art and Back Pain

The wonderful thing about Universal Martial Art is that it is a highly effective exercise that anyone can do. Since back pain affects almost 80% of all people at some time, Universal Martial Art is the perfect activity for the general public. Universal Martial Art helps to alleviate most of the risks to back pain. Done regularly, Universal Martial Art will certainly combat obesity, strengthen the bones, muscles, and tendons, and combat stress and anxiety. The components that make up the Universal Martial Art system are safe, relaxing, and enjoyable. Therefore, no one who practices Universal Martial Art will have a reason to revert to a sedentary lifestyle. The large flowing movements in Universal Martial Art combined with the Universal Martial Art stretch go a long way toward preventing occurrences or severity of back pain and treating back pain when it occurs. This makes Universal Martial Art the ideal treatment for back pain occurrences. For the effective treatment and prevention of back pain, those areas support the back-need movement and stimulation. That is why bed rest is a poor prescription for back pain. Someone once said, "An ounce of prevention is worth a pound of cure." The investment one makes into taking Universal Martial Art classes pales in significance to the cost of dealing with constant back pain. Loss of production, loss of wages, and loss of time can all be averted with just a few hours a week of Universal Martial Art training. Considering new studies in back pain treatment, Universal Martial Art is just what the doctors have ordered.

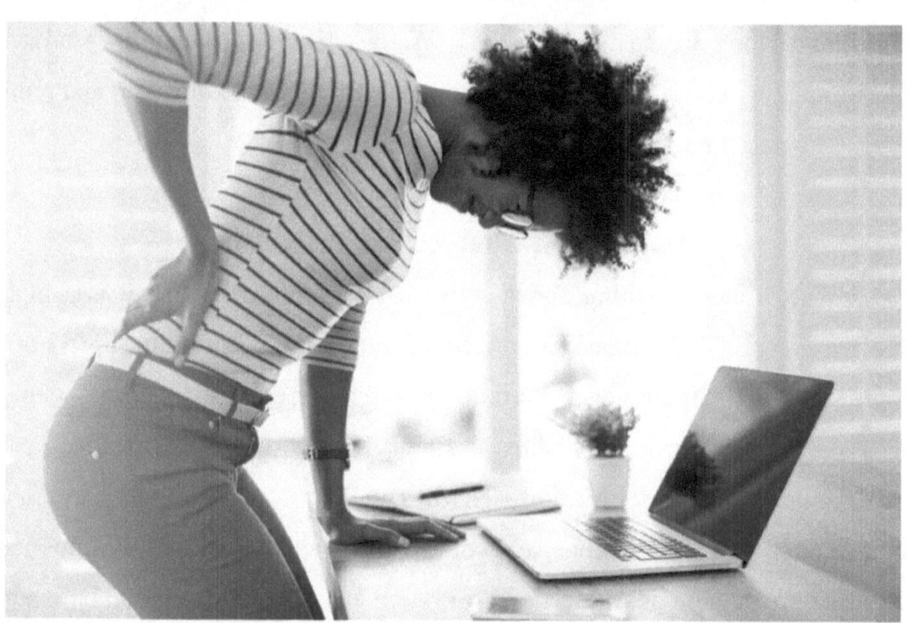

Personal Training and Osteoporosis

Osteoporosis means "porous bones." It is a progressive disease in which bones become brittle and thin. This condition ultimately leads to fractures or broken bones. These fractures or breaks often occur in the spine and hip. Hip fractures or breaks result in hospitalization. Fractures or cracks in the spine result in loss of height and severe back pain. Osteoporosis is a "silent disease" because most people who have it do not know it until a bone break. Osteoporosis is a threat to about 44 million people, of which 80% are women.

During the younger years up to about 30 years old, the human body produces new bone faster than the body can absorb the old bone. After the age of 30, this process starts to reverse. Bone is absorbed more quickly than new bone can be added. The bone becomes thin and will break even with the slightest injury. A person is more likely to develop osteoporosis if they did not reach ideal bone mass (density) during the early years. Osteoporosis is a very preventable disease.

When done in the early years, building bone density is like putting money in the bank for retirement. When an older person retires, the amount of money they receive diminishes related to the amount of money they spend. Therefore, they must have money in the reserve to compensate for those lean years. This is true where our bones are concerned. People should spend their young years building up bone mass while they can. Bones are living tissue that is constantly changing. They are always in the process of building up and breaking down. Osteoporosis results when the bone breaks down faster than it can be built up. Bone density usually reaches peak strength at 25 years. After that, to slow down the progress of bone degeneration, one needs a calcium-rich diet and weight-bearing (resistance training) exercises. Also, eliminating junk foods and soda will go a long way to help maintain good calcium levels in the bones. The body does not produce calcium. A person must get it in through their diet. When the body does not get enough calcium, it must break down the bone to get it. Again, especially in the early years, diets lacking calcium and not enough exercise play a significant role in the development of osteoporosis.

Osteoporosis and Exercise

The best way to prevent osteoporosis by strengthening the bones is to exercise regularly. Even a person who has been diagnosed with osteoporosis can exercise to help maintain the bone mass that they have. Exercise is not just to build endurance and muscle. Exercise helps to build strong bones (mass or density). To build strong bones, an exercise program must have three elements. First, there must be a weight-bearing exercise. This is composed of an exercise that holds the body up using the feet and legs. Activities like dancing, stair climbing, walking, and hiking are examples of weight-bearing exercises. Cycling and many aerobic exercise machines at health clubs are not weight-bearing activities. Second, there must be resistance training. Resistance training consists of pushing weight or lifting against weight. This is to build strong, lean muscle. Also, studies have shown that resistance exercises help to increase bone density and reduce the risk of fractures. Third, flexibility training needs to be a part of the exercise regimen for injury prevention.

Universal Martial Art and Osteoporosis

Universal Martial Art provides the best overall approach toward the prevention of osteoporosis. It has all the elements necessary to help combat this silent disease. Universal Martial Art kicks, patterns, and speed drills are weight-bearing exercises. Target training provides essential resistance training. The

Universal Martial Art stretches offer the necessary flexibility training. With an early start in Universal Martial Art, children get a head start in preventing the onset of osteoporosis. The gradual increase of stress that comes with the rise in difficulty and intensity of the kicks and punches in Universal Martial Art helps the body and skeletal system adapt. It adapts by getting stronger. However, with too much stress, as in competitive sports activities, the bones and muscles will break down. Suppose scientific research and health experts agree that the elements necessary to combat and even relieve the effects of osteoporosis are effective exercises. In that case, Universal Martial Art needs to be recognized as a leader in helping to prevent and treat such a debilitating, degenerative disease. It contains in its system all the elements necessary to provide an effective defense against threats of conflict and effective protection against threats to optimal health.

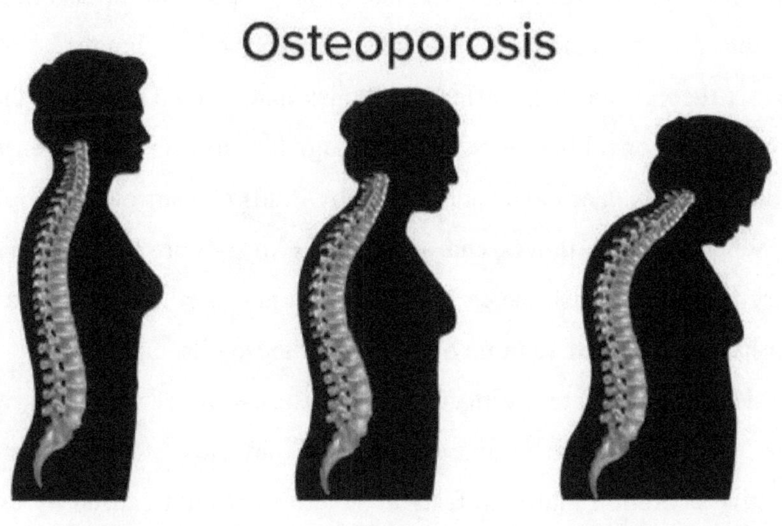

Personal Training and Arthritis

Arthritis is a general term encompassing about 100 different conditions affecting 46 million adults and 300,000 children in the United States. The most common form of arthritis is osteoarthritis, affecting people over 60 years old. Of the 100 different conditions, there is one common thread. Such affects the musculoskeletal system, particularly where two bones meet (joint). The symptoms of arthritis are pain, inflammation, stiffness, and even cartilage damage. The consequence of this damage is a joint weakness which can complicate everyday activities such as walking, grasping, brushing teeth, etc. Arthritis is the leading cause of disability in America and costs the U.S. Economy 124 million dollars because of medical expenses, lost wages, and lost production.

Arthritis means joint inflammation. This inflammation comes from stiffness and pain that often spreads to other body parts. As this condition occurs, the cartilage breaks down, muscles weaken, and bones deform, becoming more problematic for the sufferer. The sufferer experiences limited movement. Cartilage is the cushion that buffers the bones that meet. This keeps the bones from wearing out or rubbing together. Cartilage has no veins or nerves and thus has no blood supply. Cartilage is nourished by fluids that surround the joints.

When a person moves with a full range of motion, this helps bring the necessary fluids to nourish the cartilage. Also, it is crucial to maintain a healthy diet that has a balance of suitable oils. Without these oils, cartilage will become dry and deteriorate. There are many different forms of arthritis. The two most common are osteoarthritis and rheumatoid arthritis. Osteoarthritis is a degenerative condition that manifests in severe joint pain caused by abnormal cartilage wearing. With this pain comes stiffness and muscle weakness which result in further damage. This condition stems from either poor posture or overuse and overtraining. Many competitive athletes developed this condition because of the stress and strain of sports competition. People who are obese tend to develop this condition because of the extra weight born by the joints. Rheumatoid Arthritis is a disease associated with an autoimmune disorder. The immune system loses its ability to distinguish between healthy and unhealthy cells. The immune system attacks healthy tissue, resulting in problems affecting bones, joints, and body organs.

Arthritis and Exercise

Exercise helps to relieve the symptoms of arthritis. Depending on where arthritis has developed, the proper training will help increase flexibility, reduce soreness and stiffness, strengthen the muscles, and promote weight loss. A person who has arthritis must receive instruction in proper exercise and motion. He must be careful not to engage in wasted movement. There are three types of exercise that the sufferer needs to perform regularly and moderately to ensure the most significant benefit: range of motion exercises that consist of stretching and flexibility training, strength training consisting of weights and other resistance type exercises, and aerobic and anaerobic exercises that consist of workouts that help to elevate the heart rate. Moderate, consistent exercise will result in a minimal risk of osteoarthritis. However, studies have shown that an exercise that is high in intensity and impacts joints, such as football and soccer, is a cause of arthritis. To help prevent and treat arthritis, an ideal exercise program needs to be in place.

Universal Martial Art and Arthritis

The Universal Martial Art program provides everything necessary to help prevent and treat arthritis. Universal Martial Art's large movements help supply nutrients and oils needed to keep cartilage healthy. The Universal Martial Art stretch helps to increase range of motion and proper posture. The Universal Martial Art patterns and speed drills provide a great aerobic exercise when done with moderate intensity. This will help to improve circulation and aid in weight loss. Universal Martial Art target training provides resistance and aids in muscle strength and development. Muscle strength helps to prevent stiffness and to relieve joint pain. Universal Martial Art provides a comprehensive development plan to help anyone of any age prevent and treat degenerative disease. Universal Martial Art is the best program with highly trained instructors to guide and support students toward optimal health, using scientific principles to achieve a person's fitness goals. There are many exercise programs; however, Universal Martial Art is superior to them all. Even other martial arts systems do not have the components that make Universal Martial Art unique and effective. Anyone interested in improving his health and preventing the onslaught of degenerative conditions such as arthritis will do well to enter a Universal Martial Art program or use a personal trainer that has expertise in this form of martial art.

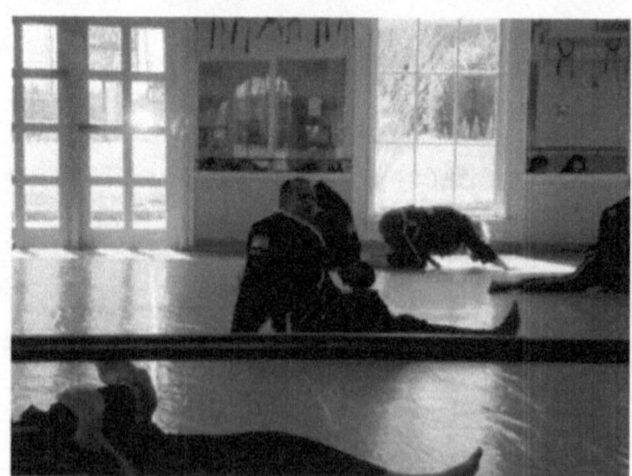

Personal Training and Fibromyalgia

Fibromyalgia is a syndrome that medical experts once diagnosed as being in a person's head. This is because the medical experts could not assess any problems with lab tests. Fibromyalgia is an arthritis-related condition characterized by pain in the muscles, ligaments, and tendons. Such pain has propelled people into lives of misery and, in many cases, has led to depression. The condition is debilitating. Recent studies, however, have shown that Fibromyalgia does exist and affects about 2% of the population in the United States. It wasn't until 1990 that doctors in rheumatology recognized Fibromyalgia as an actual condition. They determined that those who displayed the following symptoms had Fibromyalgia. The symptoms include:

- Widespread pain in 11 to 18 points on both sides of the body, usually around the trunk, that lasts at least three months
- Fatigue that interferes with normal daily activities
- Disruption in sleep routine
- Morning stiffness that lasts at least an hour
- Headaches and even migraines
- Irritable bowel syndrome
- Difficulty concentrating and even memory loss
- Depression

Because the symptoms of Fibromyalgia can be mistaken for other conditions, doctors must rule out those other conditions to properly diagnose Fibromyalgia.

No one is certain as to what causes Fibromyalgia. Among some theories is that those with fibromyalgia have a lower tolerance to pain due to abnormalities in neurons, neurotransmitters, and even the autonomic nervous system. One thing that medical experts agree upon is that stress tends to trigger the onset of Fibromyalgia. Those at risk for the conditions seem to be mostly women and those with a family history of Fibromyalgia. Also, those with rheumatoid conditions are at risk for Fibromyalgia. Of all the theories developed from studies as to Fibromyalgia causes stress is the common thread.

Exercise and Fibromyalgia

Since there is no cure or medicine (other than to provide temporary relief from pain), the best thing anyone can do in treating fibromyalgia is exercise. There may be some pain associated with the exercise at first. However, exercise must be regular for effective exercise and noticeable results. The exercise should consist of gentle stretching and low to moderate aerobic activity. Such activities would include walking, jogging, cycling, and swimming. Many people living with Fibromyalgia reduce their physical activity because of their pain. They promote lower levels of stamina and decrease strength and flexibility. Regular exercise can help to relieve pain, maintain cardiovascular health, increase the blood flow to muscles and even combat sleep disorders. The person will be able to perform daily activities with more energy and ease. The body of medical research contends that exercise is the best treatment for Fibromyalgia. A carefully controlled exercise program can improve the quality of a sufferer's life by reducing pain, enhancing mood, and improving physical function. Exercise helps improve the quality of sleep and minimize the risks of depression. The sufferer needs to participate in the appropriate kind of exercise program that will maximize his health benefits. An exercise routine that is too intense may do more damage than help. The sufferer must avoid over-exertion as such will add to his woes.

Universal Martial Art and Fibromyalgia

Since the best remedy to combat Fibromyalgia is exercise, the ultimate exercise is Universal Martial Art. The components of Universal Martial Art are essential in helping relieve Fibromyalgia symptoms. The stretching helps to stimulate the muscles, tendons, and ligaments to allow one to move more freely and painlessly. In conjunction with the large movements in the patterns, the stretch helps relieve stress and ease the severity of pain. Because the UMA class is free of sparring and competition, students can concentrate on their performance and train in a more positive atmosphere. Such helps minimize the risk of depression and lack of motivation with many exercise programs. UMA has highly trained and knowledgeable instructors who will monitor the pace and quality of the class to maximize the benefits. The students will have greater flexibility, stamina, and strength. They will have their spirits lifted in that the Universal Martial Art exercise will help to release certain chemicals in the body to provide that sense of wellbeing. If exercise is the most practical and effective way to treat Fibromyalgia, there can be no better exercise than Universal Martial Art.

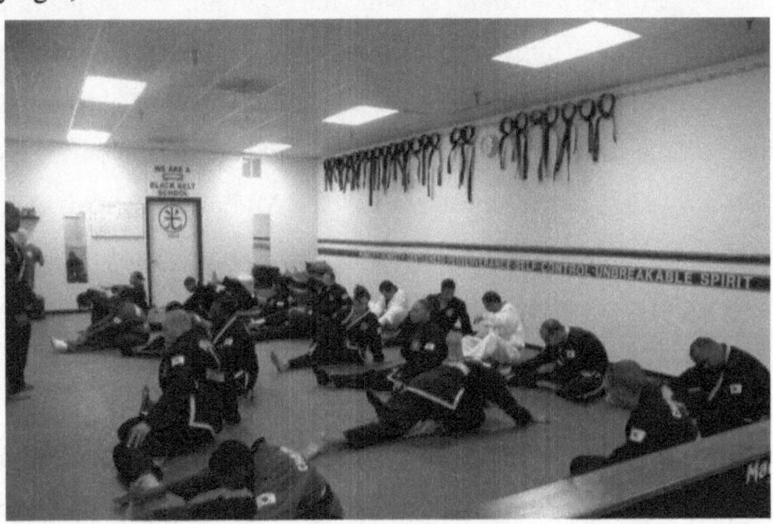

Personal Training and Multiple Sclerosis

Multiple Sclerosis is a chronic, debilitating, and disabling disease that attacks the central nervous system. Health experts consider Multiple Sclerosis to be an autoimmune disease. The body's defense system attacks myelin, the fatty tissue that surrounds and protects the nerve fibers in the central nervous system. The attack leaves these nerve fibers scarred (Sclerosis). This affects the impulses that travel to the brain, resulting in various symptoms that may differ from one person to another. Some symptoms include numbness, blindness, loss of motor skills, sexual function, and paralysis.

The exact cause of Multiple Sclerosis is unknown. However, medical experts have narrowed its causes to four areas. First, the immunologic cause is when abnormalities in the immune system are apparent. Second, the environmental cause is when certain world areas have higher disease rates. In the case of Multiple Sclerosis, studies show that those that lived closer to the equator had fewer incidences of Multiple Sclerosis. They suggest that those living near the equator absorb more vitamin D with the sunlight, which helps promote immune system health. Third, genetics play a role in determining who acquires this disease. While Multiple Sclerosis is not hereditary, having a parent or sibling with Multiple Sclerosis increases the risk of developing it. Fourth, infectious causes are constantly under consideration for Multiple Sclerosis. Childhood infections may have an impact on whether a person acquires Multiple Sclerosis. Approximately 400,000 people in the United States have Multiple Sclerosis (MS).

The medical profession diagnoses 200 new cases every week. I have had the opportunity to serve a friend in need for almost a year. He had a very aggressive case of Multiple Sclerosis. At first, he was able to eat and shower for himself. In just a few short months, he had to have a feeding tube, could no longer talk, and had sponge baths. Within a year, he died. I have another good friend with Multiple Sclerosis that was not as aggressive. He is not able to walk because of muscle stiffness. I believe if he had been more diligent in maintaining a regular exercise regimen, his MS would not have progressed to the point it did. Instead, he ate poorly, increased his weight, and added to his woes. Now he is being cared for in a nursing home.

Multiple Sclerosis and Exercise

Moderate, regular exercise is beneficial for overall health and wellness. For the MS sufferer, exercise is crucial. Even a little exercise will help retain flexibility, balance, and a sense of well-being. Exercise will add to cardiovascular fitness and regulate appetite, bowel movement, and sleep. MS sufferers understand the importance of relieving stress. Some suggest that stress only complicates and worsens symptoms of Multiple Sclerosis. Exercise is an essential activity for the relief of stress. The MS sufferer must choose a careful and effective exercise to maximize the benefit. The sufferer must be careful not to get overheated as heat bothers the MS sufferer. A 1996 study of Multiple Sclerosis patients who exercised showed greater cardiovascular health, bladder and bowel function, improved strength, and lessened fatigue and depression. Many sufferers of MS refuse to exercise because they believe that such would cause relapses of symptoms. This is a myth, however. Even a person in advanced stages of MS can benefit from exercise. While exercising, body temperature may rise, indicating relapse, but such will dissipate after about 35 minutes when exercise has concluded.

Universal Martial Art and Multiple Sclerosis

Universal Martial Art is a well-regulated exercise system that will aid in achieving cardiovascular fitness, muscle strength, and overall well-being. At the same time, Universal Martial Art is beneficial for relieving stress. Universal Martial Art movements are not stressful, and the practitioner can perform them at a suitable pace. Because of the connection, Universal Martial Art has with the central nervous system (CNS) can help stimulate the central nervous system as no other exercise can. This will help to avoid deterioration of the nerve fibers. Universal Martial Art is a progressive system that continuously challenges the CNS. The Universal Martial Art stretch and lower abdominal breathing will help stimulate the immune system. This makes Universal Martial Art the ideal treatment and prevention of Multiple Sclerosis. One primary concern for people living with Multiple Sclerosis is the risk of overdoing it with exercise. Universal Martial Art is ideal because it is a relatively gentle exercise, unlike competitive sports activities and other forms of martial arts. The components of Universal Martial Art all work together to provide a complete exercise program for the individual whose aim is long-term health. With consistent, regular, and moderate exercise, even the sufferer of autoimmune disease can lead a complete, satisfying, healthy life.

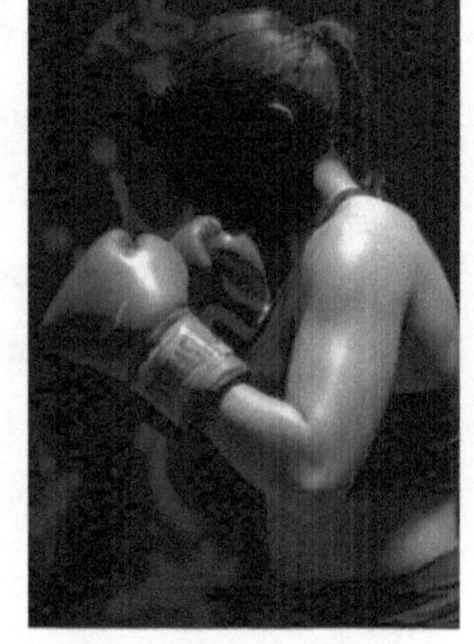

MS sufferers will serve themselves well by utilizing a personal trainer that can develop an exercise program for such sufferers. A personal trainer who knows the symptomology of MS and understands how to adequately temper exercise routines will prove to be an asset in the MS sufferer's lifestyle management.

Personal Training and Mental and Character Development

A quality personal trainer should be able to offer a total wellness package that will deliver optimal health benefits. Personal training and lifestyle management must consider the well-being of the client's mind and mental conditioning. While it is beyond the personal trainer's scope to treat mental conditions, it is within the trainer's scope to develop exercises to condition the mind and develop a strong character. The body cannot attain optimal health when the mind and inner character are not what they ought to be.

It is suitable for developing and maintaining the right mind when going through life. Positive thinking (optimism) is a tremendous benefit towards achieving good health. Improving and developing one's character will help to ensure a healthy mindset. This module is an essential element in achieving optimal health as a man of God. From a biblical perspective, the right frame of mind and upstanding character go a long way to promoting a healthy body. *"Pleasant words are like a honeycomb, sweetness to the soul and health to the bones"* (Pro. 16:24). Being positive and having peace of mind and spirit work wonders for the body. *"A sound heart is life to the body, but envy is rottenness to the bones"* (Pro. 14:30). A person lacking in character is at risk for physical decadence and disease. Add to this the fact that he affects even his mental health and peace of mind. *"The wicked flee when no one pursues, but the righteous are as bold as a lion"* (Pro. 28:1). The person who does not possess a depth of character is terrorized from within because of his constant accuser (conscience). He loses rest, worry overcomes him, and eventually, he becomes sick.

> *Why should you be stricken again? You will revolt more and more. The whole head is sick, and the whole heart faints. From the sole of the foot*

even to the head, there is no soundness in it but wounds and bruises and
putrefying sores; they have not been closed or bound up or soothed with
ointment (Isa. 1:5-6).

A personal trainer should provide the tools necessary to achieve a strong mind and character. If personal trainers only focused on the physical components of training, the training would have missed the mark on promoting optimal health. Personal training must focus on the total person if the person is to achieve optimal health. Even the Lord Himself knew of the benefits of concentrating upon the whole person (mind-mental, body-physical, soul-spiritual and social, well-being). *"And Jesus increased in **wisdom (strength of mind)** and **stature (strength of body), and in favor with God (spiritually) and men (socially)"** (strength of character)* (Luke 2:52).

The Science behind Proper Mental Conditioning

People who suffer from anxiety and stress put themselves at risk for heart disease and defects in the immune system. Studies have shown that anger and hostility in people have led to calcification of the arteries, leading to heart attacks. Grief and depression tend to lead to poor health. David had depression and sadness that led to his poor health. David wrote:

I am troubled, I am bowed down greatly; I go mourning all the day long.
For my loins are full of inflammation, and there is no soundness in my
flesh. I am feeble and severely broken; I groan because of the turmoil
of my heart . . . My heart pants, my strength fails me; as for the light of
my eyes, it also has gone from me (Psa. 38:6-8,10).

Any poor or negative emotional state puts the body in a position to accumulate acid. Other than in the stomach, acid should not be prevalent anywhere else in the body. Science calls this excess accumulation of acid in the body **acidosis**. This condition is a precursor to many debilitating diseases. A person whose diet is full of junk food and constantly stressed, i.e., emotional or overtraining, is a prime candidate for acidosis. Even a person who maintains a healthy diet yet possesses a negative mental attitude puts himself at risk. To combat this problem, one must have a positive mental attitude. He needs to find peace, love, and joy in his life. *"A merry heart does good, like medicine, but a broken spirit dries the bones"* (Pro. 17:22).

Exercise is a great contributor to good mental health. Through exercise, the brain releases endorphins (a mood-altering chemical) that assist in enabling a person's belief system (confidence/hope), thus strengthening the person's state of mind. Just exercising is not enough, however. A person must be aware of his exercise environment. Studies have shown that a person that exercises in the company of others is healthier than a person that exercises alone. Our Creator designed man to interact socially. To be healthy physically and mentally, people need people. *"And the LORD God said, 'It is not good that the man should be alone'"* (Gen. 2:18). Companionship and camaraderie are necessary for proper human development.

> *Two are better than one, because they have a good reward for their labor. For, if they fall, one will lift up his companion. But woe to him who is alone when he falls, for he has no one to help him up. Again, if two lie down together, they will keep warm; but how can one be warm alone? Though another may overpower one, two can withstand him. And a threefold cord is not quickly broken* (Ecc. 4:9-12).

Universal Martial Art and Mental Conditioning

Universal Martial Art helps to develop the mind through its martial art program. Because it is a powerful and effective martial art, the student builds his confidence because he learns to perform the Universal Martial Art techniques correctly. He is confident in his training as he sees his body respond to the effects of exercise. All this comes about while he trains in a positive atmosphere. The student becomes less stressed and more positive in his outlook. Because there isn't any competition, the harmful elements of a competitive spirit, i.e., envy, anger, jealousy, strife, hostility, and sadness, are gone.

> *What leads to strife (discord and feuds) and how do conflicts (quarrels and fights) originate among you? Do they not arise from your sensual desires that are ever warring in your bodily members? You are jealous and covet [what others have], and your desires go unfulfilled; [so] you become murderers. [To hate is to murder as far as your hearts are concerned.] You burn with envy and anger and cannot obtain [the gratification, the contentment, and the happiness that you seek], so you fight and war* (James 4:1-2 Amplified Version).

Working with fellow students in Universal Martial Art contributes to the mood-enhancing effects that bring peace, joy, and happiness when conditioning the mind. A tremendous support system in Universal Martial Art and a family environment are everything necessary to promote a positive mental outlook.

Universal Martial Art and Character Development

A person's Character helps to shape his destiny. For believers in God, such helps shape a person's eternal destiny. Nevertheless, by understanding the

Adult Pledge, Children's Promise, and Universal Martial Art Principles, the student will arm himself with the tools necessary to develop that exemplary character. The ability to achieve is crucial for building confidence and character. People will never know they have achieved anything without first setting positive goals. To achieve the goals that one has set, he must commit and discipline himself to the task. Every journey has its challenges, pitfalls, and obstacles.

A student can overcome these only with inner resolve and determination. To temper the power and skill of Universal Martial Art, the student must have a sense of right or ought. He cannot be an out-of-control weapon. He must be a person of integrity, especially if he is to interact with people from all occupations. Friendly relationships are vital for overall good health. Therefore, we must promote them. Our aim should never be to harm. In striving to promote friendly relationships, we seek to avoid conflict. We use what we learn for self-defense purposes only. As children develop character, they will learn to possess a winning attitude that exudes confidence. They will be mindful that they are still children who need able guidance and role models in their lives. They learn to respect that authority. They know to be responsible and true to themselves. They learn politeness and good manners. They learn respect for others and their safety. Universal Martial Art principles facilitate further character development to help deal with others and challenges that come their way.

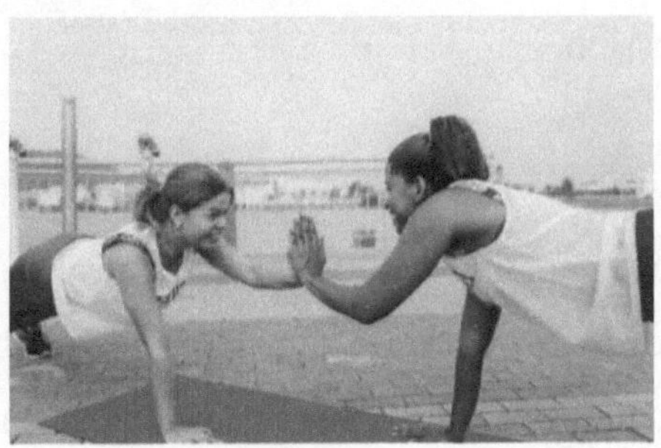

Personal Training and Depression

Nearly 19 million people over the age of 18 suffer from depression. It is one of the significant causes of suicide between 10 and 24 years old. For the second year in a row, the mortality rate in the United States has increased due to overdose and suicide, which is a direct result of some depression. Depression is a treatable condition. What is depression? Everyone experiences depression because of life's events (death, disappointment, sickness, etc.). Derivations of depression can be endogenous (from within – genetic, physical pain, chemical imbalances) or neurotic (reaction to events or circumstance – death, heartbreak, etc.). Depression is a sad mood that exceeds the average intensity and duration of sadness and grief. Such often leads to an inability or unwillingness to function in the regular usual manner. Depression symptoms are not only reflected in the person's moods, thoughts, and feelings but also may affect physical behaviors (appetite, sleep, libido, crying, etc.)

Depression can increase the risk of other debilitating diseases such as hypertension, asthma, and even HIV. Many therapists desire to treat depression with pills or electroconvulsive therapy. Many experts agree that stressful environments or circumstances trigger depression in most individuals in their diagnosis. Stress is the brain's way of alerting the body that there is trouble. The person who is always stressed (troubled, anxious, scared, hurt) is a leading candidate for depression.

Depression and Exercise

The key to combating depression is controlling stress, and the key to managing stress is exercise. Exercise helps to eliminate the adrenaline that affects stress levels. With practice, the brain releases beta-endorphins that act as an antidepressant in some or anti-anxiety in others. Either way, exercise provides a mood-enhancing benefit that contributes to most people's general sense of well-being. Besides the physical benefits of exercising in combating depression and stress, participating in and focusing on the activity helps take a person's mind off what troubles him. He also achieves a sense of accomplishment that helps to raise his mood to a more positive tilt. Exercise helps combat a person's anxiety or depression, improve their self-image, and create a buffer to protect them from stress. Exercise improves the person's cardiovascular system, contributes to neurological development and growth, and bolsters the immune system to help the person cope better physically when stress-related events do come.

Universal Martial Art and Depression

The type of exercise that one derives from performing Universal Martial Art is conducive to promoting optimal health. Universal Martial Art techniques are based upon scientific principles that consider natural and optimal body performance. The components of Universal Martial Art are ideal for helping maximize a person's overall physical well-being. The movements are not harsh or stressful but somewhat relaxed. The student of Universal Martial Art must take the time to focus and think about the movements to perform them correctly. This affects his central nervous system, stimulating neural development. The focus on proper breathing helps bolster the immune system, while stretching contributes to good blood flow and stress-relieving chemicals. The student practices Universal Martial Art in a class setting that helps to enrich the person's social interaction. This promotes good emotional health in that he has a sense of belonging, develops camaraderie, and provides a caring and encouraging environment for all students.

Because of the design of Universal Martial Art, it is the ideal exercise to combat such ills as depression and stress.

Developing a Healthy Brain

Depression has its basis in the brain of the individual. The complexity of the brain allows it to affect the body's performance. The mind can trigger such because of its belief system. *"As a man thinketh in his heart, so is he"* (Pro. 23:7). As with all other parts of his body, a person must exercise and strengthen his brain. The brain must sense human interaction and love. Loneliness, detachment, and rejection contribute to bouts of depression. Universal Martial Art classes go a long way toward resolving this crisis of the mind. A proper diet is necessary for a healthy brain. High cholesterol and obesity are leading contributors to dementia. As previously noted, exercise is vital for developing a healthy brain. The brain must be challenged. It must think about new things. With Universal Martial Art, the student constantly learns new techniques and patterns to stimulate the mind and body. Universal Martial Art is exciting and easy to learn. Students train in a non-combative, safe, and stimulating environment. With too much challenge, stress levels increase. This is not the problem with Universal Martial Art. The principles of Universal Martial Art will go a long way toward helping to improve a person's character and lift his spirits.

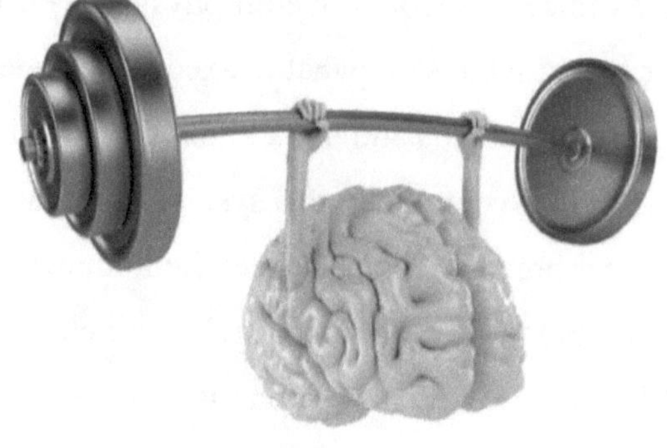

Universal Martial Art is the ideal exercise for both mind and body. It is a natural antidepressant. With the support of like-minded people in Universal Martial Art, a person can arm himself with all he needs to combat such afflictions like depression and stress. Personal training must consider this in any program a trainer develops.

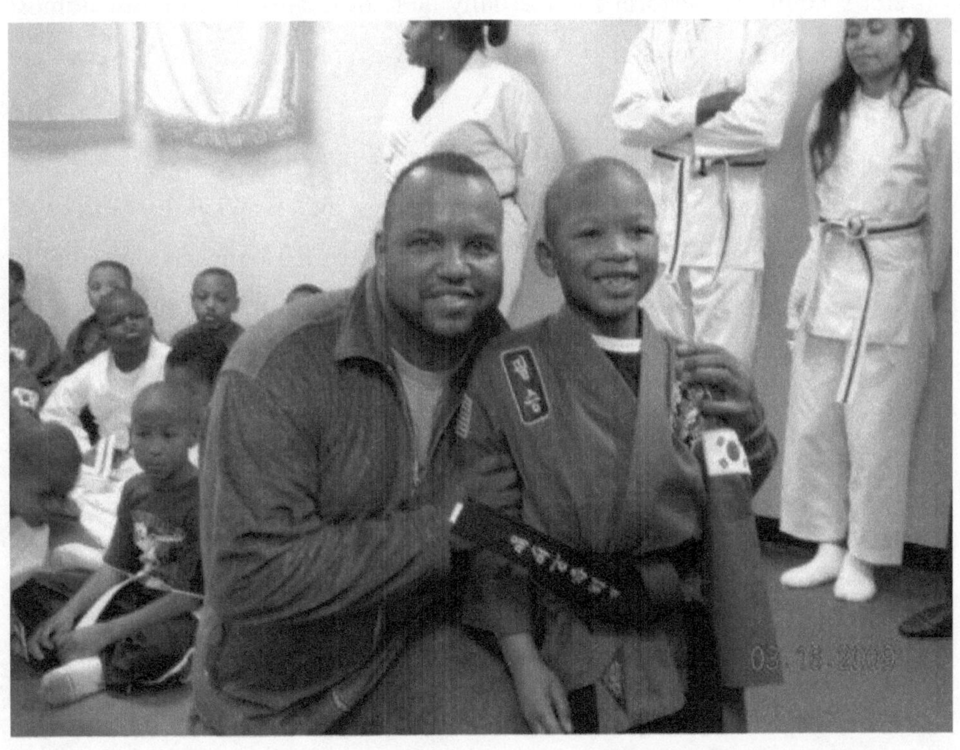

Personal Training and Alzheimer's

Alzheimer's was first diagnosed by Dr. Alios Alzheimer when he noticed changes in the brain tissue of a woman who died from a mysterious brain illness. He saw clumps and tangled fibers that now are indications of Alzheimer's disease. Alzheimer's is a type of dementia. Dementia is a brain disorder that affects the sufferer's ability to perform routine daily activities. This disease affects most people over 60 years of age. Nearly 5 million people in the United States are affected.

Medical experts have not been able to pinpoint an actual cause for Alzheimer's. There is no cure for Alzheimer's either. What happens with Alzheimer's is that nerve cells die in those areas of the brain that are vital to memory and mental abilities. This debilitating illness certainly diminishes the quality of a person's life, leading to depression. While scientists do not know a single cause of Alzheimer's, certain factors increase the risks. Age is the primary risk factor for the cause of Alzheimer's. Every five years, people over the age of 60 living with Alzheimer's double. Another risk factor is family history. Some scientists believe that genetics is a factor in whether a person develops Alzheimer's. Some scientists found that the risk factors for heart disease and stroke may also increase the risk for Alzheimer's. People are living with Alzheimer's, at first, experience memory loss.

As the disease progresses, they begin to lose the ability to remember how to do basic tasks. They forget names and may even wander away. They become aggressive and panic-stricken. What is interesting about Alzheimer's is that it is not a normal part of the process of aging. It is not something that everyone may eventually get when they get older. Head trauma has also been linked to

Alzheimer's. Even several studies have shown that those with limited education had higher incidents of Alzheimer's.

Exercise and Alzheimer's

Studies have shown that exercise helps to relieve the symptoms of dementia. A University of Washington study suggests that exercise helps to reduce the risk of Alzheimer's by 40%. The study has even shown that exercise helps delay the onset of Alzheimer's in those who began to exhibit symptoms. Exercise lowers cholesterol and blood pressure and increases blood and oxygen flow. In addition, exercise helps to reduce the risks associated with heart disease. Research suggests that exercise benefits the person living with Alzheimer's in the same way it does anyone else. For the person living with Alzheimer's, exercise can treat and reduce depression and give the sufferer a sense of well-being. Exercise has even helped to improve physical functioning. Some experts agree that exercise is not enough to prevent Alzheimer's. They have a six-point approach that they recommend to avoid Alzheimer's. This six-point approach includes exercise, diet, vitamin supplements, brain stimulation, an active social life, and consistent spiritual practice.

Universal Martial Art and Alzheimer's

The six-point approach to preventing Alzheimer's is a novel and reasonable approach. However, there is no such six-point approach that a person can get at a store or in a gym or health club. Aside from diet and nutritional supplements, Universal Martial Art provides a complete regimen for what a person needs to aid in the prevention of Alzheimer's. The ten components of Universal Martial Art are essential to combat the onset of Alzheimer's. Universal

Martial Art provides exercise that helps to improve cardiovascular health, lower blood pressure, and improve overall wellbeing. It provides an atmosphere that assures a nurturing social environment. The movements are more complex and sophisticated than walking, jogging, and cycling. Such provides challenge and stimulation to mind and body at every level in the Universal Martial Art system. The Character Development component offers a detailed analysis of a person's mental fitness development. It develops our human character. The principles of Universal Martial Art help to enforce the spiritual aspect of an individual in a way that makes him a productive, moral, and civil citizen in his home and community. Such helps to improve the relationships one has with others. The practitioner will feel good about and be happy with his or herself, fulfilling the golden text, *"Love thy neighbor, as thyself"* (Matt. 22:39)

Experts may not have a silver bullet in combating the onset of Alzheimer's. Yet, Universal Martial Art, when practiced regularly, will go a long way in gaining the upper hand in that fight. Anyone who seeks to improve the quality of his life through such will certainly ensure that they maintain the proper diet and nutritional balance in their life, thus achieving the six-pronged approach toward the prevention and treatment of Alzheimer's.

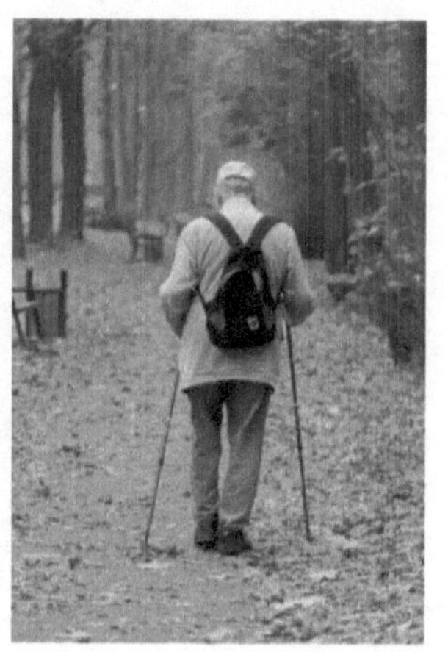

Personal Training and Parkinson's Disease

Parkinson's is a disorder that affects nerve cells or neurons in the part of the brain (basal ganglia) that controls muscle movement. James Parkinson first identified it in 1817 as "Shaking Palsy." Parkinson's costs the U.S. 5.6 billion dollars annually. It usually affects people over 50 years of age. The normal motor function relies on Dopamine, a chemical that the neurons help to produce. Dopamine sends the signals that coordinate a person's movements. When Neurons die or are abnormal in the way they function, diminished dopamine production is the apparent result. The medical community is at odds about what causes the harm to these cells. There are four significant symptoms of Parkinson's disease.

First, there are tremors. A person will have uncontrollable trembling in the hands, legs, jaw, and face. Second, the sufferer will experience stiffness and rigidity in the trunk and legs. Third, he will experience slowness in movement. Fourth, the sufferer may experience imbalance and a lack of coordination. The sufferer may have trouble walking, talking, chewing, and performing simple tasks as the disease progresses. Presently, no blood or lab work can aid in diagnosing Parkinson's.

The only thing doctors can do is rule out other diseases. Parkinson's can lead to disturbances in mood, sleep, reaction time and dementia, and depression. Parkinson's disease has no discernible cause. Some rare reasons are genetics, head trauma, toxins, and drugs. Those who suffer head trauma were four times more likely to develop Parkinson's. One interesting theory about the cause of Parkinson's, which still holds, is the existence of free radicals (which contribute to cell destruction). Oxidation usually attacks and destroys tissue; cell destruction is a part of the process. There is no cure for Parkinson's disease. Some medical experts treat the symptoms with drugs. There are at least nine kinds of medications used to treat different types of symptoms of Parkinson's. Some sufferers have held out hope of a political and scientific solution to this problem. Michael J. Fox has brought attention to this disease with his testimony before congress. He calls for embryonic stem cell research, which has proved quite controversial.

Exercise and Parkinson's

There isn't a study that I know suggesting that exercise can cure Parkinson's disease; this does not mean that no benefit can be had from regular exercise. Regular exercise in people with Parkinson's has improved motor skills, trunk rotation, hand-eye coordination, stability, muscle strength, and non-motor skills. One compelling study highlighting the benefits of exercise in people living with Parkinson's is one out of Osaka Medical School in Japan. About 80% of people living with Parkinson's in the study lived longer lives because of the benefits of exercise. Those with Parkinson's can sharpen their mental and physical capabilities.

Universal Martial Art and Parkinson's

Universal Martial Art (UMA) is the exercise for the 21st century and beyond. In the medical studies about Parkinson's, one such theoretical cause stood out. The idea that free radicals may be the culprits behind the onset of Parkinson's needs to be further explored. Free radicals are usually connected with the start of cancer. They are molecules of oxygen that have lost an electron. Free radicals result from oxidation, which is generally a destructive force in nature. Free radicals are the body's terrorists attacking neighboring cells, tissue, and organs, searching for the coveted electron. Since Parkinson's links with cell destruction in the brain that affects the delivery of dopamine, anything that can combat and eliminate free radicals in the body is paramount. The ideal way to stop such destruction is to ensure that one is engaged in regular, moderate levels of fitness training. Exercise helps boost antioxidant production, which helps curb free radical production. UMA is a highly controlled and regulated exercise and self-defense system. It considers intensity, frequency, duration of exercise, the release of chemicals from the brain under certain circumstances, human anatomy, and body functions. In other words, every scientific consideration has been implemented in the design and formation of the Universal Martial Art system, making it the ideal exercise in combating and eliminating free radicals. The UMA components such as stretching, patterns, speed drills, defense drills, warm-up, cool-down, and resistance training combined to address every facet of optimal human health. Even Parkinson's sufferers, if they benefit from exercise, will be sure to benefit from Universal Martial Art. The Universal Martial Art movements' challenge and complexity help promote cellular growth. It helps to promote

balance, strength, fitness, focus, and mental wellbeing. With the high cost of medications that serve only to mask symptoms, Universal Martial Art is not only ideal but practical.

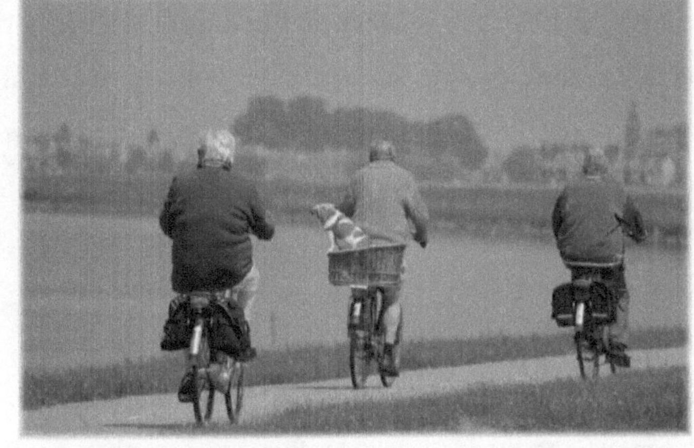

Nutrition and Recommended Daily Intake

An accurate journal of foods consumed will go a long way to determine what type of nutritional intake a person needs to meet their Recommended Daily Intake (RDI). One place to look to determine what an individual's RDI should be is choosemyplate.gov. This is the government's daily recommendation. We will consider other elements such as caloric intake, Macronutrient distribution, etc. While exercise is essential for overall fitness, proper nutrition ensures energy levels are needed to promote physical activity and provide the right nutrients for exercise recovery and muscle growth.

Macronutrient Intake Ranges

Consuming macronutrients within the RDI ranges is crucial because too little or too much can impact a person's health, the difference between preventing disease and degenerative conditions that put one at risk of obtaining disease. Too little protein can affect resistance to diseases, poor muscle growth, and body function in the growth years. Too much protein, especially from animal meat, can adversely affect the kidneys and be responsible for uric acid build-up, causing gout. Because carbohydrates are the primary source of fuel for the body, a diet with too few carbohydrates will result in sluggishness, one becoming mentally drained, bad breath, and even poor kidney function. Those that do not consume enough fats in their diet put themselves at risk of suffering nutritional deficiency. This is because fats help the body to absorb the nutrients it needs. Also, low fat can hinder hormone production. Add to that the fact that not enough fat can impact growth and overall body health.

Intake of Carbohydrates, Proteins, and Fats

Carbohydrates always come in the form of sugars, starches, and fibers. One can find these in fruits, vegetables, grains, and milk. They provide an immediate energy source to the body and are essential for a healthy diet. Carbohydrates are macronutrients. Macronutrients are how the body gets its energy. They come in carbohydrates, fats, and proteins, which the body converts for energy and bodybuilding. The body uses carbohydrates for fuel first as they are not as complex as fats and proteins. Fats and proteins take more time to convert into glucose. Because they are easily converted to energy, Carbohydrates are necessary for the body's daily function. The brain is especially needy for glucose for proper operation. Proteins are not the most efficient source of fuel for the brain, and fats do not break down to serve the brain well either. The brain works 24/7, thus requiring around 130 grams of carbohydrates to function correctly. The number of carbohydrates that the brain needs accounts for 40%-65% of the RDI of calories. So, diets such as the Keto diet are not the most effective for optimal health and fitness.

Fats are a macronutrient: Trans fats, saturated fats, monounsaturated fats, and polyunsaturated fats. Trans fats are the absolute worst in that they are processed fats from good fats. They go through a hydrogenation process to allow good fats to harden. Trans fats are in margarine, store-baked goods, potato chips, and restaurant fried foods. The purpose is to increase the shelf life of foods. Trans fats are harmful in that they lower HDL and raise LDL. Foods that contain partially hydrogenated fats or oils should be avoided. Saturated fats are fats that become solid at room temperature. Sources of saturated fats are animal meat, dairy, and coconut oil. While there are some benefits from saturated fats, RDI should not contain more than 6% of its calories from saturated fat.

Monounsaturated fats are those that one can find in olive oil and avocados. These fats do not harden at room temperature and are very heart-healthy. There are not any restrictions on their consumption. Polyunsaturated fats are fats that the human body does not produce.

Thus, we must find adequate sources of polyunsaturated fats as a part of our RDI. Polyunsaturated fats are canola oil, corn oil, salmon, mackerel, tuna, soybeans, flaxseeds, and walnuts. These fats help to promote cardiovascular fitness. They help to improve one's cholesterol profile and improve muscular efficiency. Fats are necessary as a part of one's RDI because of all the reasons and because they help the body absorb essential vitamins.

Additionally, fats act as an energy reserve. The body processes carbohydrates initially for energy. After about 20 minutes, the body begins to tap into the fat resources for energy.

Another critical element for proper body function is protein. Protein is also a macronutrient that can be either complete or incomplete. To be complete, the protein needs to have all nine amino acids. Most plant proteins are incomplete proteins but can provide the complete proteins needed by the body, combined with other plants. Sources of complete proteins are eggs, meat, fish, and dairy. This is important because the body is constantly growing or renewing itself. The amino acids help in muscle growth and tissue repair. Also, these help to build the body's immune system. Besides meat and dairy, proteins can come in nuts and beans, and some vegetables. When broken down, protein helps to fuel muscle, boost the immune system, increase metabolism, and make one feel satiated. A person's body weight is 15% protein and needs an RDI of 10%-35% of calories in protein. Those who recommend and those who live on high protein diets to exclude carbohydrates do not consider the health risks that come from such a nutritional imbalance. While one may see an immediate drop in weight, the long-term effects on the body can be detrimental. Carbs are an essential macronutrient. Following the RDI for macronutrients is a necessary and wise decision one must embrace for overall health and fitness.

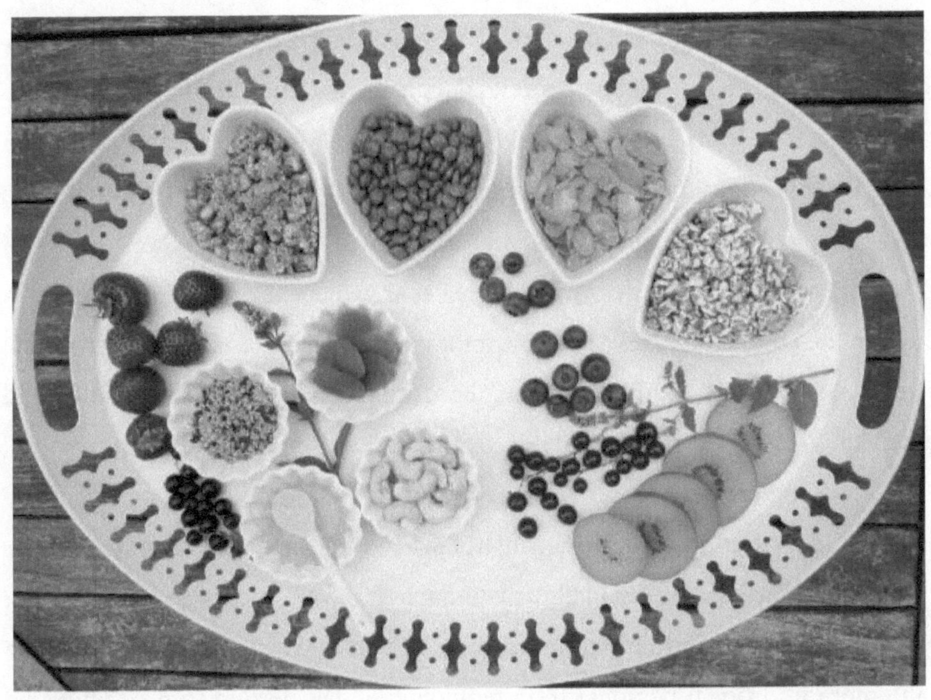

Conclusion

There is an adage in the Bible from Luke 4:23, *"Physician, health thyself."* As a personal trainer, I will do all I can to ensure that I am an example of health and fitness for the clients I train. Especially as a 57-year young person, I hope to inspire people my age or approaching my age.

I have chosen to incorporate Universal Martial Art training into my programs. My services are more beneficial than any health club. If I had to choose between a health club and Universal Martial Art, Universal Martial Art is the choice without question. Unless a person is part of a health club that is everywhere, he may not have a place to train when he travels. The students of Universal Martial Art can do what they learn anywhere they go if there is not a school in the area. Universal Martial Art may not be as big as some health clubs; however, there is no health club out there that compares to the quality and effectiveness of Universal Martial Art, the martial art for everyone.

I am determined to provide the most effective training program for my clients. I am blessed to be a Master instructor and international Faculty member in Universal Martial Art. This helps distinguish me from most personal trainers. I will incorporate this into my training programs for my clients, along with some of the more traditional personal training elements that pertain to resistance and strength training. Incorporating Universal Martial Art into the personal training program is key to an enjoyable, satisfying and effective training experience. The whole idea is to manage the quality of one's life better. My approach is to provide the client with the most effective and safe methods for achieving optimal health. And Universal Martial Art does just that. When personal trainers employ the right tools to ensure this outcome, those that hire those trainers will be much appreciative.

As a personal trainer, I will do the necessary assessments to determine functionality and medical clearance for exercise. I will also observe and monitor the movements of the exercise to ensure that they are safe and effective while being done correctly. Because I am a personal trainer and Universal Martial Art instructor, I can help prevent, manage, and relieve the symptoms from the onset of various degenerative medical conditions. I will develop and monitor the fitness routines I deliver to my clients to ensure they are safe and not too intense. Everyone deserves the opportunity to enjoy a certain quality of life that will not lead to pain and depression.

My training philosophy embraces the essential elements necessary to improve the quality of a person's life. Physically, I incorporate Universal Martial Art training which addresses every aspect of a person to develop their body right (flexibility, cardiovascular fitness, strength). However, *"Bodily exercise profits a little, but godliness is profitable for all things having promise of the life that now is and the life that is to come [destiny]"* (1 Tim. 4:8). We must also develop our minds and character if we want to be complete people in optimal health and improve the quality of our lives. Then and only then will we be able to fulfill our destiny. *"Who is the man who desires life, and loves many days, that he may see good? Keep your tongue from evil, and your lips from speaking deceit. Depart from evil and do good; seek peace and pursue it"* (Ps 34:12-14). Is it any wonder why men have termed Universal Martial Art "the martial art for life?" Therefore, I am confident and happy to incorporate martial arts, particularly Universal Martial Art, into personal training.

I hope you have found the information in this book beneficial and rewarding. Please follow up by visiting my web pages: **www.cslmpt62.com** and

www.smartacademyuma.com. Please take advantage of any personal training programs I have to offer.

I look forward to working with you in the future.

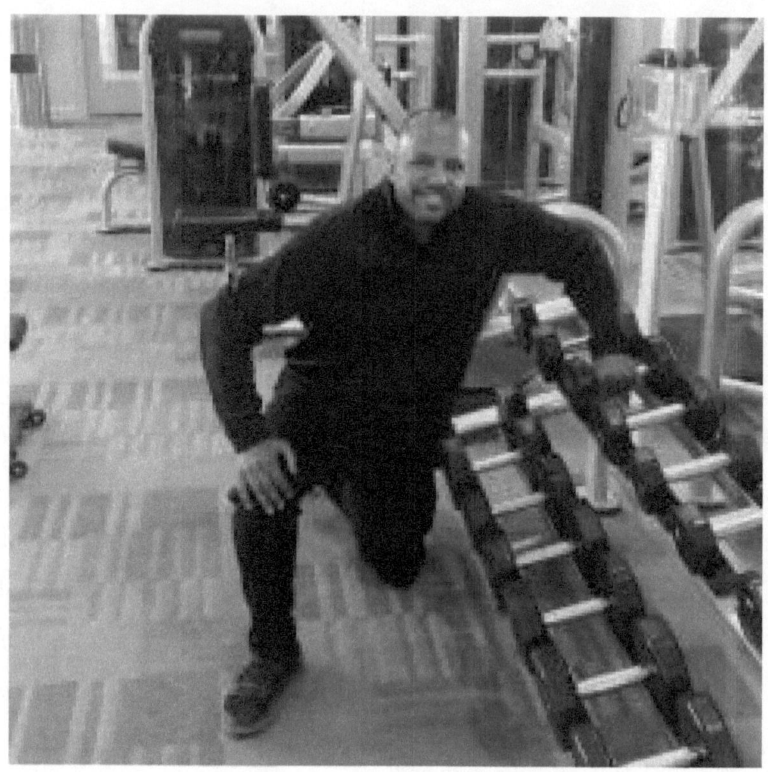

References

Baillie, H. W., & Casey, T. K. (2004). Is human nature obsolete? genetics, bioengineering, and the future of the human condition.

Bjarnadottir, Addahttps (2019, July 10). 9 Reasons Why Obesity is Not Just a Choice. Retrieved from //www.healthline.com/nutrition/9-reasons-obesity-is-not-a-choice

Crowley, C., & Lodge, H. S. (2007). *Younger Next Year: Live Strong, Fit, and Sexy-Until You're 80 and Beyond*. Workman Publishing.

De Lau, L. M., & Breteler, M. M. (2006). Epidemiology of Parkinson's disease. *The Lancet Neurology*, *5*(6), 525-535.

Doyle, C., Kushi, L. H., Byers, T., Courneya, K. S., Demark-Wahnefried, W., Grant, B., & Andrews, K. S. (2006). Nutrition and physical activity during and after cancer treatment: an American Cancer Society guide for informed choices. *CA: a cancer journal for clinicians*, *56* (6), 323-353.

Ellenbecker, T. S., & Davies, G. J. (2001). *Closed kinetic chain exercise: a comprehensive guide to multiple joint exercise*. Human Kinetics.

Guide to Clinical Trials and Studies at the UW (2019). Retrieved from //depts.washington.edu/mbwc/adrc/page/clinical-trials

Hannaford, C. (1995). *Smart moves: Why learning is not all in your head*. Great Ocean Publishers, Inc., 1823 N. Lincoln St., Arlington, VA 22207-3746 (paperback: ISBN-0-915556-27-8, $15.95; hardback: ISBN-0-915556-26-X, $24.95).

Harkcom, T. M., Lampman, R. M., Banwell, B. F., & Castor, C. W. (1985). Therapeutic value of graded aerobic exercise training in rheumatoid arthritis. *Arthritis & Rheumatism: Official Journal of the American College of Rheumatology*, *28*(1), 32-39.

Khachaturian, Z. S. (1985). Diagnosis of Alzheimer's disease. *Archives of neurology*, *42*(11), 1097-1105.

Kumanyika, S., Jeffery, R. W., Morabia, A., Ritenbaugh, C., & Antipatis, V. J. (2002). Obesity prevention: the case for action. *International journal of obesity*, *26*(3), 425.

Kushi, L. H., Doyle, C., McCullough, M., Rock, C. L., Demark-Wahnefried, W., Bandera, E. V. ... & American Cancer Society 2010 Nutrition and Physical Activity Guidelines Advisory Committee. (2012). American Cancer Society Guidelines on nutrition and physical activity for cancer prevention: reducing cancer risk with healthy food choices and physical activity. *CA: a cancer journal for clinicians*, *62*(1), 30-67.

Lawrence, R. C., Felson, D. T., Helmick, C. G., Arnold, L. M., Choi, H., Deyo, R. A., ... & Jordan, J. M. (2008). Estimates of the prevalence of arthritis and other rheumatic conditions in the United States: Part II. *Arthritis & Rheumatism, 58*(1), 26-35.

Legge, A. How to Estimate Your Maintenace Calories. *Complete Human Performance.*

McDonald, W. I., Compston, A., Edan, G., Goodkin, D., Hartung, H. P., Lublin, F. D., ... & Sandberg-Wollheim, M. (2001). Recommended diagnostic criteria for multiple sclerosis: guidelines from the International Panel on the diagnosis of multiple sclerosis. *Annals of Neurology: Official Journal of the American Neurological Association and the Child Neurology Society, 50*(1), 121-127.

Myers, J. (2003). Exercise and cardiovascular health. *Circulation, 107*(1), e2-e5.

Nigg, B. M., MacIntosh, B. R., & Mester, J. (2000). *Biomechanics and biology of movement.* Human Kinetics.

O'Sullivan, P. B., Phyty, G. D. M., Twomey, L. T., & Allison, G. T. (1997). Evaluation of specific stabilizing exercise in treating chronic low back pain with radiologic diagnosis of spondylolysis or spondylolisthesis. *Spine, 22*(24), 2959-2967.

Obesity and Overwight. (2016 June 13). Retrieved from //www.cdc.gov/nchs/fastats/obesity-overweight.htm

Pan, X. R., Li, G. W., Hu, Y. H., Wang, J. X., Yang, W. Y., An, Z. X., ... & Jiang, X. G. (1997). Effects of diet and exercise in preventing NIDDM in people with impaired glucose tolerance: the Da Qing IGT and Diabetes Study. *Diabetes care, 20*(4), 537-544.

Salmon, P. (2001). A unifying theory is the effects of physical exercise on anxiety, depression, and sensitivity to stress. *Clinical psychology review, 21*(1), 33-61.

Sawka, M. N., Burke, L. M., Eichner, E. R., Maughan, R. J., Montain, S. J., & Stachenfeld, N. S. (2007). American College of Sports Medicine position stand. Exercise and fluid replacement. *Medicine and science in sports and exercise, 39*(2), 377-390.

White, L. J., & Dressendorfer, R. H. (2004). Exercise and multiple sclerosis. *Sports medicine, 34*(15), 1077-1100.

Wilkins, Isaac (2007, November 5). The Pros and Cons of Group Exercise. Retrieved from //ezinearticles.com/?The-Pros-and-Cons-of-Group-Exercise&id=818623.

Wilmore, J. H., Costill, D. L., & Kenney, W. L. (1994). *Physiology of sport and exercise* (Vol. 524). Champaign, IL: Human kinetics.

Woodward, T. W. (2009). A review of the effects of martial arts practice on health. *Wisconsin Medical Journal (WMJ), 108*(1), 40.

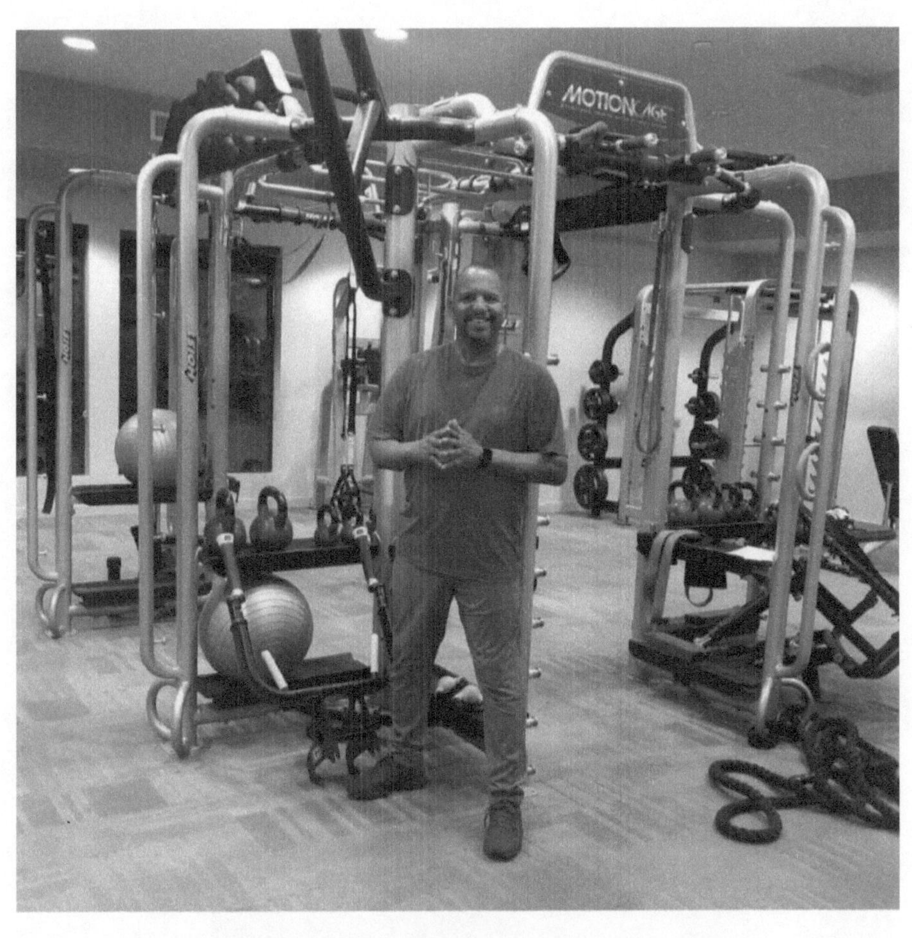

Charles "Charlie" Spence, Jr.

ACE Certified Personal Trainer

6th Degree Black Belt

International Master Instructor